THE BABY BOOMER'S MOTIVATIONAL GUIDE TO WEIGHT LOSS

By Scott "Q" Marcus and Cindy Marcus

Cover Art by Niki Key

Acknowledgments

Scott's List:

With so much gratitude, our cups runneth over--

There are many people who go into making a book possible. And we wanted to make sure this amazing group got their due. Let's start with Scott's list:

Cynthia MacGregor and our publishing house. Cynthia not only grabbed on to our idea but ran with it like a "bat out of hell." (Couldn't resist one more last reference...) Also to her for calling me "sweetie" every time I talk to her (an expression my mother used all the time) and of course for shepherding us through this process.

Niki Key, whose wonderful cover design really captured the spirit of our book and brought huge, broad smiles to our faces.

Russ Riddle for his generous donation of time.

Richard Borough and the Master-Mind Alliance, Jessica Pettitt, Rich DiGirolamo, Gerry O' Brien, Eliz Greene, and Thom Singer, who told me over and over to speak to what I know and love. It took me a long time to hear it; thanks for shouting.

The editors of the newspapers that have run my weekly column for over a decade and the thousands and thousands of loyal and dedicated folks who attend my meetings and presentations and follow me on line. I am honored beyond expression for the support over the years.

Daniel and Brandon, my sons, who think I can do almost anything. May I someday feel on the inside the way they see me on the outside.

My wife, the love of my life, the light in the darkness, my soul mate through centuries past and yet to come, Mary Ann Testagrossa, who has stood by me through every crazy idea I've had, supporting me when I needed it and being my guard rails when I go off track. There are no words deep enough to express what I feel for you.

...and of course, my little sister and co-writer. The faith you showed in me by nurturing my seedling into a million roses has allowed me to live what I never dreamed. This isn't your brother talking, but you're a phenomenal editor and writer and I'm thrilled we got to work together. What will we wear on *Ellen*?

And now Cindy's list:

Cynthia (Cyn) MacGregor, editor extraordinaire, and now lifelong friend. Thanks for your joy, smiles, and enthusiasm.

My male muses whom I love beyond measure:

Flip Kobler. The best husband/partner/friend EVER! And thanks for all your help on this book. As always, you make the work and the journey so much better.

Finn Kobler, my "eye apple" and the inspiration for all things wonderful in my life. You continue to inspire me to be the best person I can be.

Dennis Poore, my "other husband" who is always there when I need you, sharing the adventure.

Brad Green, my brother from another mother. Editor, believer, and sushi buddy.

Ann Harris. My BFF. You give me the answers, even when I'm not asking…and sometimes don't want them, but you are always, always a rock, and an angel in cowgirl clothing.

The cowgirls, Linda and Michelle, thanks for celebrating my ups…and downs.

The Plotkin clan: Jeff, Tami, Joel, Ellie. You are so much more than family.

The amazing publishing house, PrimeTime. Aach! I'm so excited about our relationship. I hope it grows and grows and grows…

SCBWI. And all my peeps there. But special shout out to Laurisa, Mary, Cheryl and Karen.

And then, of course, my big bro, Scott. My friend, my hero, my funny man. I adore you. Thanks for trusting me with your baby. I love that we get to do this together.

FOR OUR M&Ms

Mary Ann, Mom and My Men

WHY DID YOU PICK UP THIS BOOK?

Have you been trying to lose weight since Gilligan was stranded on his island? Did you look at John Travolta's pure white suit in *Saturday Night Fever* and think, "Black is so much more thinning?" Did you want to wear hip-huggers, but all you could fit into was a muu-muu?

Then, you've picked up the right book.

Let us introduce ourselves.

SCOTT: Cindy, you go first.

CINDY (in that bubbly, full-of-life, exciting manner that is her): Uh, really? Okay, cool. What should I say?

SCOTT: Just say who you are.

CINDY: Hi. I'm Cindy!

SCOTT: Perfect. You did really well.

CINDY: Aren't you going to introduce yourself?

SCOTT: Sure, I'm Scott.

You see, we're a brother-and-sister team who has been on the front lines of the diet wars since Julie Andrews and Dick Van Dyke danced with a cast of animated penguins. We've tried it all, from Atkins to Zumba, and just like you, we've had our ups and downs—literally, on the scale.

However, we have now both been at our "ideal" weights for a long time. And we can and *will* help *you* get there, too.

You ready?

Bitchin'. Let's get started.

Like us, you've probably tried: pills, powders, and all food concoctions not found in nature. You've awakened before the sun to power-walk, jog, run. You know the fat, fiber, and carb content of every food on five continents. You've low-carb'd, high protein'd and even been anti-gluten. Yet you still haven't kept the weight off.

Let's face it: Dieting blows! (Like we have to tell you that.)

That's 'cause "diets" don't work. "Diets" are complex systems to a very simple formula: Eat less; move more. When you really bring it down to brass tacks, losing weight isn't complicated; it's actually really simple: Keep your mouth shut and your feet moving. That's it.

So, why do our plates remain overloaded and our pants too tight, and why do the numbers on the scale continue to rise?

What's that about? What's missing?

Guess what? You're not missing anything. You're awesome. The problem is you've been asking yourself the wrong question. As the Moody Blues crooned, "Why do we never get an answer when we're knocking on the door with a thousand million questions…?"

The key is to make sure you're asking the *right* questions. Once you do that, you will find your way to that wonderfully fit body you've always wanted.

We're here to give you the questions. You already have the answers.

WHY THIS BOOK?

Why will this approach work when others have not?

Wise question, Grasshopper.

The answer is that virtually every diet out there focuses on the three Cs: carbs, calories, and calisthenics. Oh sure, each diet brands its program differently, but when boiled down to the basics, it's the same tired advice couched in a bright new package: eat less, move more.

They can phrase it however they wish. They can wrap it up in all manner of fancy-schmancy, quasi-scientific jargon, but they're still telling you what you already know: Shut your mouth and keep your feet moving.

Those way cool new "diets" forget one major thing: You are already an expert on what to eat and how to eat it. You could teach everyone from Jack LaLanne to Richard Simmons a thing or two about a thing or two. You've been there, done that. Been on Johnny Carson. Had the t-shirts made…, (You get the picture)

What this book will do for you that is different is *focus on the cause, not the symptom.* Identify that reason, come up with a plan to deal with it, and you're gonna stop all the yo-yo dieting and keep it off. For good.

Warning, Will Robinson, warning: This next sentence might seem counter-intuitive, but it's true. In order to lose weight—and keep it off—eating right and exercising regularly are *not* your first steps.

Wait. That's so important for you to grok that we're going to repeat it:

Eating well and regular exercise are *not* the first steps to a healthier lifestyle. Rather, they are the end result of a long chain of thoughts, feelings, and beliefs you have about yourself.

Let's explain:

You're alone in the house after everyone has gone to bed. It's ten, ten-thirty, and the end of a really crappy day. Your boss has hit you with a ton of unexpected work that's going to dig into your weekend plans. (Isn't it time to retire yet?) Your teenage son has been in a mood since 2012. The dog just peed on the floor. And you are done. Just done—with everything.

Okay, so what are you going to do?

Choice One: You do the healthy thing and go to bed.

Choice Two: Since nothing has gone the way you hoped today, you might as well just march into the kitchen and dig into that half a gallon of cookie-dough ice cream that's been calling your name.

So what did you do? Choice One? (Good job. Pass Go and collect $200.)

Yeah, right.

Most likely you went for what was behind door number two. Of course you would. It's been a really bad day, you need something to comfort yourself, and in that moment, as you are facing the fridge with all those thoughts and feelings roiling around in your gut, you know that ice cream will not let you down. Its perfect, creamy goodness understands.

You see? Eating has nothing to do with knowing all the right things to do. Paying attention to "what your body is telling you" or "hunger signs" or "the best carbs" isn't going to stop you that you from eating that box of Twinkies, any more than knowing your term project was going to be due at the end of the year would cause you to start writing it on day one.

That's 'cause being "thin" has nothing to do with *knowing* what to do. It's about identifying the triggers that drive you to that binge-starve food-fest that you get involved in *in spite of knowing what to do,* and redirecting those triggers.

Once you see the patterns, and then know and understand its triggers, you can implement simple, easy-to-do, (dare we even say) fun activities that will help you stay fit. You will actually be able to beat back that mean old food demon that has controlled you for far too long and live that healthy lifestyle you've dreamed about for so long.

So to that end, unlike any other "diet tomes," this book will not tell you that you need to cut back your calories, eat fewer carbs, or exercise more. No nifty recipes will you find among these pages.

We know you get what to do. You know the basics of weight loss. You know that you need to cut back and eat healthier. You know that increasing activity is important. You sure as heck don't need us—or anyone else—wagging our/their finger at you and scolding you about what you've tried to do for most of your life. The advice within these pages is unlike that in other books because it will help you understand—and change—that frustrating lose-gain cycle in a way that others have not. It will ask the right questions.

This book will help you think about why you do what you do. And when you engage that big, beautiful brain of yours, you'll be able to choose what you want to do to be happier, healthier, and even thinner.

We will help you get past what's been holding you back and actually move toward the results you've longed for since you sucked in your belly to squeeze into that first pair of bell-bottoms.

WHY US?

In other words, what gives us the authority to write a book like this?

As we stated, we're a baby boomer brother and sister who have spent most of our lives battling weight. We come from a long line of pleasantly plump people who have also fought weight all their lives.

WHY, ME? - SCOTT

I spent the first thirty-nine years of my life fat, entering the world at 9 pounds, 14 ounces and then going uphill from there, weighing ten more pounds for every year of my life. When I was five, I weighed 50 pounds; when I was ten, I crossed 100. I remember as if it were yesterday the humiliation of shopping in the "husky" section. By the time I reached my teens, however, I really ballooned, tipping the scale at 237 pounds. I was the boy girls said had "a nice face and a good personality." Boys teased me mercilessly; I was challenged to flagpole fights with regularity, simply because of my weight. Needless to say, I hit my teen years desperate to take off the weight.

While I was growing up, our parents took me to doctors whose only solution was giving me those 1,000-calorie-a-day diets on countless purple-mimeographed pages. "Eat only from this list, and make sure it's 1,000 calories a day or less," they would say. And I would nod my head, agreeing to whatever the doc said...for a day, maybe two—until that next mean taunt. Then off I'd slip, putting back on whatever weight I'd lost—and then some.

Something changed when I turned sixteen. Our parents, who were also obese, began attending meetings provided by a major weight loss organization. (We can't tell you what that is, but its name rhymes with Nate Notchers.) They came home with a food scale and scads of booklets, diaries, and other groovy info.

I, being a science nerd (right down to the tape across the bridge of my glasses), was fascinated by all the nifty gizmos and gadgets needed to lose my weight. I liked that I needed to attend a weigh-in every week. It was helpful that members supported me. And it didn't hurt that I was the only teen in a roomful of "old" women (in their thirties and forties) who embraced and supported me. I lost almost 100 pounds by the time I turned seventeen!

Alas, it didn't stick…

I gained back most of my weight a few years later and, as a DJ in northern California, playing the hits like "In the year 2525" and "One of These Nights," once again decided to return to what worked. This time I dropped 80 pounds and achieved goal weight for the second time, becoming one of very few male lecturers for that company, certainly one of the youngest.

Know what? It still didn't stick.

For a decade, I'd lose and gain the same few pounds, yet all the while trending upward. Finally, on my thirty-ninth birthday, at 250 pounds with a 44-inch waist, in a failing marriage, suffering from chest pains, backaches, and a life spiraling out of control, I hit rock bottom. After everyone left my birthday party and my family went to bed, I got down on my knees in the kitchen and scarfed the leftover birthday cake—from the garbage.

Horrified at what I was doing, I returned to the fold, determined to never again feel so humiliated and degraded, promising to be "fit, fun, and fiscally sound by forty." Three hundred sixty four days later, one day before my fortieth birthday, I tipped the scales at my correct weight.

That was September 27, 1994.

WHY DID IT STICK THIS TIME?

Therapy. A whole lot of "self-work." And the decision *not* to focus on losing weight but rather to understand why I did this to myself—why *we* do this to ourselves. I realized I needed to treat the causes rather than the symptoms. Now, as a professional speaker, consultant, and trainer who has spoken all over the country on the topic of changing habits, I've analyzed and studied what makes successful dieters successful. And I'm going to share what I've learned with you.

Right now, though, let's let Cindy introduce herself....

WHY ME? - CINDY

Hi. It's me. Cindy. So, "Hi!"

Well, like Scott, I loved to eat, and at twelve years old, I was as tall as I was wide. Shy and fat and ethnic looking, I didn't exactly have boys—or even friends—beating down my door. Desperate to wear halter tops and hot pants like the really hip girls, I too jumped on the Nate Notchers diet train. And at thirteen, (drum roll please) I hit goal weight! And I was actually able to buy clothes from the 5, 7, 9, clothing store. Jeff Kykendall, the very cute basketball player in my middle school, actually noticed me in my adorable maxi dress and asked me to dance—at a dance, you understand. (He didn't just walk up to me in the halls and say "Let's dance." I mean he had good taste, but he wasn't crazy.)

But Jeff asking me to dance meant I'd arrived. Me? Me! I knew forever forward I would now be skinny and stylin'. The world was my oyster..... Not.

The weight loss didn't stick.

And because I believe in full commitment, *my* freshman fifteen became the freshman many more than fifteen. (I went to four colleges, so you do the math.)

With handsome young men once again not knocking upon my door and my fragile self-esteem disappearing rapidly, I, like my big bro, returned to the diet dance.

Off will go this weight, said I, as on came therapy and self-discovery, and all those great Me Generation things we did in the '70s.

I ate brown rice and rice cakes and wore Birkenstocks and embraced my inner Zen. I tried yoga and meditation and nicer versions of EST. I was determined to like myself.

And in the process met—cue Cupid-like angels—Flip. This handsome, green-eyed man, who looked a lot like a young David Bowie, actually loved that I had almond, deepset eyes and a strong Jewish nose. He didn't think I needed a nose job. He said, "What makes you different makes you beautiful." (I know, right? Was I lucky or what?)

Anyway—cue the very best angelic choir you can think of—we fell in love. Who needed to eat? With "passion feeding my soul" (I know it's cheesy, but hey, love will do that to you), I kept the weight off—right? No. (Sad face.)

The weight loss didn't stick....

But for a really good reason! I gave birth to my solo child, the wonderful apple of my eye and then some—Finn.

However....

I should probably be honest here. I didn't put on any weight during my pregnancy 'cause the docs thought I had gestational diabetes, when in fact, Finn was just a big, *big* baby—but I had to diet. Then after Finn was born, I breast-fed. And that is the most amazing thing 'cause you get to eat and eat and eat and you don't put on a pound.

And then Finn got colic and, believe me, you don't want to eat when your kid has colic. You want to cry and scream and yell, 'cause this beautiful, amazing thing in your arms won't stop screaming. He's got a delicate little belly, and whatever you eat when you're breast-feeding, he feels. So again, I dieted to help my baby. Of course.

Ah, and this is where the plot thickens....

So. Finn was now free of colic and onto teething. I hadn't eaten like I thought a pregnant woman was "entitled" to eat—and since I'm really good at rationalizing anything, I ate. (Mind you, at this point I was actually thinner than I had been pre-pregnancy —oy!) But I was determined to have all that chocolate and cake and chips I was "entitled" to have as a pregnant person. So I put on 13 pounds in no time.

I took it off.

And this time it stuck!

WHY DID IT STICK THIS TIME?

I learned that "successful" thin people put on weight. Really? They do. Skinny people put on weight all the time. They go up and down just like we round people. The trick is that their ups and downs are less uppy and downy than ours.

Their up and down isn't 15, 20, 80 pounds, it's 5. Maybe 7. Isn't that amazing?

I could be a successful thin person if I just didn't go past that dreaded 5 or 7 pounds!

And that's what I've done. I've kept myself to that range. Up I go. Down I go. Now, to be honest I really, really, *really* love the down. It makes me feel young and svelte and adorable, and I don't have to lie down to button my jeans.

I don't like the up. I don't. 'Cause it triggers that trigger (which we'll discuss in this book), and I'm on a downward spiral to shame.

However—and this is a big *however*—I don't beat myself up like I used to. As you will discover, the weight gain is actually a signal that something is off kilter.

And although it takes a while, the weight does come off. Until it goes back up again. But that's okay, because I adjust. You see? Staying thin is a journey—not a destination, and I think I finally get that.

WHY US?

This book is a compilation of the best lessons we've experienced, and heard, about staying motivated to take weight off and *keep it off*.

There are no scientific studies here ('cause, really, haven't you already read enough of those?). This book contains a combined total of over 100 years of being on the front line of the diet wars (yikes—are we really that old?) and *knowing what works*. We have both been leaders—and continue to be—in our weight loss tribes. We have both run the gamut of guru-led diets. And we have both have kept our weight off because we know what works. We have looked inside and understand *why* we eat. We have come up with alternatives that replace that unpleasant dessert of guilt and pounds that comes along with eating too much food.

And we are going to share those ideas with you!

So remember, this book isn't a "dieting" book.

It *is* a "learning-to-ask-the-right-questions-and-incorporate-the-answers" book. It *is* a "learning-about-what-triggers-you-to-eat-and-stopping-the-unwanted-cycle" book. It *is* a "recognizing-that-you-have-everything-you-need-to-achieve-the-life-you desire" book.

To that end, we might use the word "diet" once in a while. However, we are not talking about the starve-yourself-give-up-all-your-favorite-foods-and-eat-cling-peaches-cottage-cheese-and-one-meat-patty deprivation sessions we went through when we were young. It's a short cut for the words, "program," or "habit change." You can insert whichever you feel most comfortable with. This is your journey

So, the bottom, bottom line of all this is this book is all about building a better way to live, putting you in alignment with the *you* whom you have always had inside, and letting that *you* come out.

So let's get started....

Oops! Wait! *(Sound of Wiley Coyote screeching to a stop to avoid going over a cliff.)*

There is one last thing. And this is important.

By now, you're seeing that *The Baby Boomers Motivational Guide to Weight Loss* is written for—wait for it—Baby Boomers! Unlike our younger counterparts, we, some of us, have been dieting for fifty or sixty years. We are career dieters who are ready to retire that medal.

So, we have designed this book for you, sweet Boomer, made to fit into your life smoothly and easily. We are *you*. And we understand how busy life is at this age. So, although we are going to ask you to do some tasks, we have made them simple and easy.

Your first "task" is to make sure you have a pen as well as a notebook handy. (See how easy that was? We didn't steer you wrong did we?) It doesn't have to be expensive. But do make sure it's a color you like. You can even choose one with a design on it, like Johnnie Quest or Galactus. If you want to add in stickers and some crayons, even better! This is your journey. Do your own thing.

Whenever you pick up this book, make sure you have your nifty notebook and pen at hand. Scattered throughout these pages, there will be many times when we'll ask you to write down some thoughts—or even to play. (Just make sure you're home by dark!)

When you get to those sections, it's time to stop reading and start doing. Do whatever the book tells you to do. It's not a chore. Or a task. And please, oh please, don't make it into work. If you find you don't have time, do it later. Be kind to yourself. Believe us, we understand; but make sure to do what we ask. You won't have to show it to anyone, and no one is judging you; no teacher is grading you.

So, are you ready?

You have your notebook and pen ready?

Then let's move forward.

CHAPTER 1: WHY MAKE IT FUN?

Blah, blah, blah…. Enough talk. Time for some fun.

Think back to the game Freeze Tag. Remember? We'd all run around our yard, and the kid who was It (not the *Addams Family* Cousin Itt) would chase us and try to tap us. When that kid did, we'd have to freeze in place. Once everyone was frozen, It was free to be an Itee (or a chased kid).

Okay, we're a collective It. We have just tapped you and…"Freeze!"

Now reach for your notebook and write down the first five words that come to mind when you picture having to lose weight the old-fashioned (wrong) way, through deprivation and sacrifice. Now look at your list.

What emotions are evoked?

We'll bet dollars to donuts (yumm, donuts) that "Fun" didn't enter the list.

See? Therein lies the problem.

You might have noticed that we have used the word "fun" a few times already in context with weight loss.

(Whachu-talkin'-bout, Willis?)

It's been a feeling associated with weight loss about as often as Archie Bunker was associated with "liberal."

That's because dieting up to this point hasn't been fun.

Eating ice cream is more fun than eating celery. Chips are more fun than fat-free…well…anything. Watching *Harold and Maude* for the umpteenth time is more fun than huffing and puffing your way down the street in a jogging suit that makes your behind look like a couple of raccoons fighting in a gunny sack.

And since we—at our age—can get soooooo tired after we take care of everyone else, we *need* fun, it stands to reason that if we can make this journey more fun, it makes it more likely we'll stick to it. And the longer we stick to it, the more the odds increase that we'll see results. And you know what? Results are way righteously bitchin' far out fun!

So to that end we've scattered "fun" things throughout these pages. Some will make you laugh; others will bring out your more creative side. But they're all designed to help you be more successful by lightening your load (both figuratively and literally).

We know that not everyone will jump on this. After all, years of being overweight can generate some pretty heavy self-consciousness.

However, can we point out another side, please? First of all, aging is not for the young. Also, we believe we never truly grow up; we simply become wrinkled kids. Sure, on the outside, it seems that everything is getting hairier, softer, and closer to the ground, but on the inside, there's a small child yearning to be set free. So let's make this journey to our happy body place joyous. Therefore, we hope you'll embrace the fun in this program with three features you'll find regularly throughout these pages.

- The World According to Scott
- Let's Play
- He Said/She Said

WHY "THE WORLD ACCORDING TO SCOTT?"

CINDY: I'm going to take it from here for a few minutes. I don't want to brag about my big brother, but Scott's a funny guy. And he tells really good stories. Our mom said he was the first person to make me laugh. And he can still turn a bleak day around for me with his warm, yet slightly twisted sense of humor.

His tales from the front lines of weight loss make me giggle. And more important, his stories help me to not be so hard on myself when I falter, and to laugh at some of the ridiculous things I do and just get back up on that horse and keep going.

We've interspersed "The World According to Scott" throughout the book.

Scott's World isn't serious; it's always in good fun. You'll probably see yourself in Scott's world. I sure do. Most likely you'll nod and grin—which burns calories! (We don't know how many. But we know it does.)

WHY "LET'S PLAY?"

SCOTT: My turn now. My sister is one of the most playful, upbeat, fun people you will ever meet. She might be a Baby Boomer in years but she's a little kid in spirit and what keeps her eating on track is making sure she gets enough playtime. So we've come up with a series of games and activities for you to do that will help you to integrate the "lessons" we are sharing in a playful way.

Plus there's the fact that the people with letters after their names—doctors and such—who have done studies on learning—say that since we are all a bit visual and verbal learners, the best way to reinforce learning is with words to read and tasks to do. But it's up to you to decide how you wish to integrate the lessons in this book into your life

You're a Boomer. We know that you know what's best for you.

WHY HE SAID/ SHE SAID?

Repetition is necessary if we want to integrate change. Did you know that if you want to lose a habit you have to not do that habit-y thing for twenty-one days? Twenty-one days! So we felt it important we reiterate—in many different ways—the points we are making. Hence, He Said/She Said—a dialogue between the two of us that will recap what you have hopefully learned in the chapter.

Oh yes, as Columbo used to say, "One more thing..."

You know those negative feelings you wrote down at the start of this section? Cross 'em out! Better yet, crumple up the page and throw it away. Seriously. We'll wait. (Insert "Girl from Ipanema" on-hold music.) Consider it an act of empowerment or another blow against the empire, but they are now part of your past.

Life is already getting better. Can't you feel it?

CHAPTER 2: WHY DID WE NOT SEE THIS?

The World According to Sc⊕tt

Dear Diary,

Sunday: My backside looks like cottage cheese during an earthquake. Tomorrow I go on a diet. Here's to success!

Monday: I'll start Tuesday. We had treats in the house and had to get rid of them. In retrospect, it might have been smarter to throw them away instead of eating them, but what can you do? At least the house is clean of fatty foods, giving me a running start tomorrow. Here's to success!

Tuesday: So far, so good! No cravings. No slip-ups. We'll see how it goes after I get out of bed. I think I'm going to make it.

Wednesday: My alarm didn't go off so I didn't exercise—but I did try on five pairs of sweatpants to see which looked best. Now I'm really set for tomorrow. Watch out, world!

Thursday: The sweats weren't clean; can't exercise in dirty gym clothes, so I put that off until tomorrow. In other diet news, I got an order of fries on my way home. At first I felt bad, but then I realized potatoes are vegetables, so I got a larger order. This dieting thing isn't so hard.

Friday: Finally got to exercise! I walked to the coffee shop down the block and got a chocolate chip muffin to replace all the calories I burned. Later, the family went to a Mexican restaurant. I realized I might be eating a little much when the waiter brought a fourth basket of chips. So to compensate, I had two light beers instead of regular ones. I don't understand why people complain about diets; this is easy. You just need to think about what you do.

Saturday: What a busy day! Between running the kids around, going to the mall, and housecleaning, I'm surprised I had time to breathe. About 4:00, I realized I hadn't eaten, so I did three rounds of samples in the grocery store. The amounts they give are so little, there's no way I put on weight. Tomorrow, I get on the scale. I can't wait!

Sunday: Dieting doesn't work! I've been perfect all week and—can you believe I gained two pounds?! What's that about?! I'm going to figure out a new plan and start again tomorrow. Right now I have to go; we're late for pizza.

WHY IS LOSING WEIGHT SO HARD?

Remember the gnarly game Mousetrap? You got to build this way cool, Rube Goldberg-type contraption to try to capture your opponent's mouse. It really was the most convoluted series of cogs and wheels and gears to do a simple task. Heck, that's what Rube Goldberg was known for.

Anyway, the thing was that it worked. Gears would turn, causing balls to follow a twisty path, and in the end, a plastic guy "jumped" into a tub, and you experienced either the thrill of victory or the agony of defeat. But it did the job.

So, where are we going with this?

There's an expression: "Every system works perfectly to achieve the results it delivers."

In our case, we weren't trying to capture cheese, but we had built a perfect system to be overweight. Stated another way, you *weigh what you weigh because of systems you have built.*

You see, it's not that those of us who weigh too much are lazy, inept, or stupid. We have just—over the years—built a system that functions perfectly to *allow* us to gain weight.

We know you didn't intentionally build that system of weight gain, but build it you did. The proof is in the Jello mold each and every time you stand on the scale.

You indeed did create a successful system of eating that allowed you to put on weight.

Uncomfortable to look at it that way, isn't it? You actually created this body you are living in. You might not have meant to. But it was *you* who did do this to *you*. We know those are hard words to hear. And accept.

We've been there.

The realization that we were responsible for our own weight gain was so hard. But it was an important step in our journey. To keep the weight off, we had to own the weight we'd put on. Ironic, huh?

As difficult as it is to tell yourself, "I created this size," you must do it. And you must accept and believe it. But don't beat yourself up!

Cindy and Scott's number-one rule of weight loss (truth be told, we number all the rules "number one" so you don't have to remember the order) is "If shame and guilt were motivational, we'd all be skinny." So stop the blame. Stop the guilt. It. Does. Not. Work.

Next, back away from the pizza. *(Remember, we've been there).*

Take a deep breath and realize that you were doing the best you knew how to do at the time. In the same way you now know stuff that you didn't know as a thirty-something and didn't even know you didn't know, and now don't do that stuff 'cause you know better—you know?

In other words, you, in the past, did the best you knew how to do at that time. So instead of self-recrimination, how about...

Let's Play

We call this The Oy. And we dedicate it to our bubbie (that's grandmother, in Yiddish), Lottie.

Lottie had this expression she used whenever she was frustrated or disappointed or tired or—well, whatever negative she was feeling, she used it. And it always—*always*—made her feel better. And she passed it on to our mom, who passed it on to us. Because we like you so much, we want to give it to you.

This expression was so simple, yet so powerful it could change an entire outlook.

You wanna know what it was?

(We bet you do! Come on, admit it!—please?)

Okay, well, since you insist, we're going to tell you. The expression was—are you ready?

(This is exciting stuff. It could change your life.)

(Insert drum roll please.) The expression was....

"Oy."

Now, don't get us wrong. She didn't just *say* "Oy". She *felt* it. She *lived* it. She immersed her Russian soul in it. Bubbie would inhale deeply. And then on the out breath, as she'd say, "Oy!" her shoulders slumped, her chest caved.

When she said "Oy," it was as if she channeled over 5,000 years of Jewish suffering into her body and then let everything that had been done to her, her people. the people next door, the people down the block roll off her back all at once.

So, right now as you are acknowledging that you created this current size you inhabit, we want you to do The Oy.

Don't go all intellectual, or all grown-up on us. Don't tell yourself you'll do The Oy tomorrow or next week when you are thinner or braver or smarter, or there is no one home to hear you. Right now. Wherever you are. Take in a really deep, ginormous breath, think about all the crap that's been holding you back. Hold it in. Count. One. Two. Ready? Now exhale and sigh the word "Oy."

Oh gosh. Don't you feel better? (We feel better just thinking of you doing that.)

Now would be a good time to get out that notebook and write or color or put a sticker in it and remind yourself: 1. You did "The Oy." (fun you), and 2. You took responsibility for something you've been making excuses about all your life. You acknowledged you put on this weight. You!

Owning the body you live in is going to make such an empowering difference in your journey from here on. Once you realize that your weight gain was not a fluke of nature, and, no, you were not condemned to be heavy by Adipose, the Goddess of Cellulite, nor by your slow metabolism or your genetics or your big bones or your unsupportive family or your unfair friends or your thyroid or your....

Once you own it, you are free!

By taking ownership of this wide but very lovable thing called your body, you realize that you can make it however you wish (um, except younger, of course). Any size, shape, and even eye color you like. You now understand that you have the power to make yourself thinner or healthier or whatever "er" you wish.

Isn't that fantastic?!

When you own that you made yourself the size you are, you are free to create a new size.

And even better, since you have already been successful at creating that larger "system" think of how successful you will be at creating a smaller "system."

Now that you understand and accept that you are master of your own destiny, what you do next will matter!

Accepting responsibility—without shame (remember Rule #1)—is empowering, because once you understand you are the creator of your system, you realize that you can change that system. You are that powerful! Jeeze, we wish we were you right now!

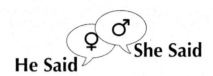

He Said **She Said**

(Since Cindy is a playwright, we thought we'd do this recap as a play)

(Cindy and Scott sit in Cindy's office. It's messy. Filled with color. Many toys fill the shelves—a five-foot plush bear, which sits on the floor, is the largest. Watsky, the bear, says nothing but beams widely at the brother and sister team.

Cindy sits at the desk, typing. Scott's in the overstuffed chair beside her. Both are working like fiends—she writing, he editing. They are pushing to meet an insane deadline.)

SCOTT:

You didn't finish this section.

CINDY:

Yeah, I did.

SCOTT:

No. You didn't. And now the chapter doesn't make sense.

CINDY:

I -ah—I was tired. Finn needed help studying. Flip needed me, can you—

(Scott stares at her. Is she kidding? Cindy shrugs, defensive.)

CINDY:

What?!

SCOTT:

This was your idea—to do a project together.

CINDY:

I've just got a lot going on—.

SCOTT:

And I don't?

(Cindy looks at Scott. She reaches out a hand. Apologetic be she. He gives her the pages.)

CINDY:

You're right. This is our book. I wanted this. It's up to me. I'll fix it.

SCOTT:

And then we'll get frozen yogurt.

CINDY:

Can we go to the place where you can put all sorts of candy and goodies on it?

SCOTT:

Like the peanut butter cups and marshmallows?

CINDY:

Oh, yeah.

SCOTT:

But no maraschino cherries. I'm trying to knock off a few pounds.

(Cindy smiles. They go back to work, she redoing the pages she didn't finish 'cause she recognizes—it's up to her.)

CHAPTER 3: WHY DO I KEEP DOING THIS?

The World According to Sc🌐tt

Why, oh why does a fierce battle rage within me each time unexpected goodies are offered?

Let me set up a scenario. I stop by Jim's office to pick up a flyer. Cake, brownies, and pie are strewn about the table in the employee lounge. He says, "We had a party in Brenda's honor today. Help yourself."

We now join the internal conversation, already in progress.

VOICE NUMBER ONE:

Wow! Look at all those goodies. Go for it!

VOICE NUMBER TWO (THE SKINNY ONE):

It's merely food, Scott! It's not like you've never had chocolate cake before. Get a grip!

V1:

But it's free. That makes it better.

V2:

It still has calories. Just because you don't pay for it doesn't mean it won't make you fat.

V1:

Ah, come on. It's just going to go to waste if I don't eat it. Think of all the starving people who would jump at a chance for this much food.

V2:

Just because it could be wasted doesn't make you the garbage disposal.

V1:

Okay, but how do you feel if you spend a whole lot of time looking for that perfect gift for our wife?

V2:

Where are you going with this?

V1:

Work with me here. So our wife opens the gift, and we can tell she's disappointed.

V2:

Bummed.

V1:

Right. And then we get all distant from her. And she pulls back. And soon we're having an argument about something that's totally unrelated, like the toothpaste cap or whether all socks go in the hamper—

V1:

What's your point?

V2:

Well, it's kind of like that, see? Jim's our friend as well as business associate, right?

V1:

Yes, so?

V2:

So, he's thinking of us by offering a chance to share in the celebration. By providing these treats, he's really saying, "We don't spend enough time together socially. I'm trying to make up for that by giving you these goodies. Please don't turn your back on me. I'm feeling very vulnerable right now."

V2:

All that is involved in this? I thought he was just being friendly.

V1:

Don't be naïve. Men aren't good at discussing emotions, so it comes out in other ways.

V2:

Well, we wouldn't want to hurt his feelings. I guess a little bit is okay.

As I reach for the plate, Jim says, "Oh yeah, I've been meaning to talk to you. You do so well watching your weight. I was hoping for a few tips."

My hand lurches to the right, and I pour a cup of coffee instead, only to hear myself reply, "It's simple, actually. Just follow your inner voice."

WHY ALL THAT SELF-DOUBT?

Why do we think we don't matter? Why wouldn't Jim or Sam or Melody want to be our friend and spend time with us? What have we done that's so bad that makes us feel so worthless we'd eat that damn cake?

Nothing!

Really!

Okay so we Boomers haven't been perfect. But, let's put it in perspective: We've weathered some pretty stern stuff. (We're not just talking about being forced to play "Bombardment" in the gym on rainy days by a sadistic P.E. teacher.) We made it through: Vietnam, gasoline lines, and the Chicago riots. We also: founded Earth Day, championed civil rights, and created the entire computer era. We're pretty right on. (Granted, we also unleashed Tiny Tim's "Tiptoe Through the Tulips" on a helpless nation, but everyone's entitled to a slip-up now and then.) So, why are we so quick to beat ourselves up for carrying around a few extra pounds?

Can we just chill out please?

Truth is we are awesome. Simply because we carry an extra pound or seven doesn't make us less than everybody else. And really, isn't the only difference between "us" and "everybody else" that our not-like is on display for everyone to see?

Picture a line of people walking down the street. Now imagine what it would be like if everyone had to have a sign announcing their hidden ick for all to view.

- A slim, attractive, fifty-three year old, graying-at-the-temples in a $1,500 suit has a placard over his head announcing: "I smoke so much that my lungs look like asphalt."

- Behind him is an eye-catching, thin woman pushing two children in a stroller. Her sign proclaims: "My credit cards are maxed out because I cannot control my spending. Also, I'm keeping it from my husband so I feel like I'm lying to him."

- A young, obviously fit man in athletic gear has a badge declaring: "I'm so afraid of personal commitment that I've cheated on every serious romantic relationship I've ever had."

- We, with our larger frames, are closing out the line with our sign, "I eat too many potato chips when I'm stressed"

Kind of puts our reasons for self-doubt in perspective, doesn't it? In the big scope of things, we aren't bad at all. We're actually kind of endearing.

WHY DO WE EAT THE WAY WE DO?

Well, let's be honest, we need to eat. That's a gimme, right? Eating is a necessary part of our existence. If we don't eat, we starve. Therefore we must eat.

And then there are eating rituals. They are part of every culture in the world. Every celebration is punctuated with food. Think about it: When was the last time you went to a party and there wasn't a snack? A wedding and there wasn't a toast? Eating is everywhere. Even at funerals.

So we're all agreed. We must eat.

The problem arises when eating becomes habitual.

What do we mean by habitual?

Well, a habit is defined as an automatic routine of behavior that we repeat regularly and without thinking, in order to make our life easier or better. The problem is that these habits have side effects, those results we don't expect.

So, let's unpack this a bit, shall we?

The key elements here are "without thinking" and "side effects."

Because eating is such an important part of our existence, it's understandable that it can become a habit. After all, we do eat three times a day—more if we're on a cruise ship—365 days a year, over how many years? That's a lot of eating!

But the issue isn't just what we eat at meals, is it? It's the eating we do without thinking, the "habitual" eating.

If we are going to attain that healthy body we long for, we're going to have to stop "habit" eating. Again: A habit is doing something *without thinking*. So we're going to have to stop eating without thinking.

If we cease the habit of unconscious eating, eating without thinking about what we're eating, we will cease putting on weight. Because if we are aware of what we're eating, and we know it's hurting us, we won't eat it anymore.

Right?

Yeah. No. We all know that simply stopping the unconscious eating thing isn't quite that simple.

WHY ISNT' LOSING WEIGHT THAT SIMPLE?

1.   We have come to associate food with comfort.

You see, when we're sad we eat. Why? To feel better. When we're angry we eat.

Why? Because who likes running around feeling P.O.'d all the time? When we're stressed? What do we do? You got it. Give us an "E!" Give us an "A". Give us a "T." Goooooo *eat*!

In reality comfort is what we seek when we grab that Dove Bar.

Food is an emotional connection to a feeling we want gone or a feeling we want back. That's another one of those really important things to learn, so we'll repeat it. Food is no longer food; it's an emotional connection to a feeling we want gone or a feeling we want back. Lock that one into the memory bank, okay?

2.   Our behaviors have side effects.

The side effect of eating to feel better is we get fat. If we want to change the side effect, we have to change the behavior.

There are people who, when they're sad, cry.   When they're angry, they exercise; when they're stressed, they meditate. (There's a clinical term for those types of people: They're called "Skinny.") Anyway, same triggers, different habit, different side effect. And we bet they can still fit in their culottes (although we're also sure they won't want to).

From "Days of our (Baby Boomer) Lives," we now take you to an example of why losing weight is not that simple.

It's another day in Boomer Land, and Bonnie Boomer is at her wits' end.

And once again, the world is dependent on her. Her aging parents are upset she isn't coming to visit—even though they refuse to move closer. Her adult daughter is having marital troubles, and she's come home. The car needs an alternator; the roof needs repair. Ugh!

Poor Bonnie is just plum exhausted.

So it's (fanfare, please), *Carbs to the rescue* (whoosh)!

A giant Hershey bar, with almonds, stands in the distance.

(Wind blows the wrapping of our Chocolate Hero, creating a cape-like effect. Bonnie swoons.)

Okay, we exaggerate. A little. But ice cream. Cake. Chips. Fraps. We also call them Junk Food. You can call them Al. (Not really.) They appear to be our best friends because they understand, and they possess the power to make our icky feelings go away. And they do it fast. And without argument.

It's no wonder we reach for comfort foods. They've always been there. And we know we can count on them in the future.

WHY CAN'T I STOP WITH JUST ONE?

When logic has taken the back seat, and emotion has the steering wheel, with her lead foot on the accelerator, the need for comfort becomes all-consuming. We need it, and we need it *now*.

We scour the kitchen or office food dispenser machine or streets looking for anything to lessen the pain. Logically, we know it won't solve the problem and, deep inside, we know we're going to feel bad later. However, as we said earlier, *knowing* what has to be done doesn't mean we'll *do* it.

Remember, we are just little children in big bodies, and when we are sad or lonely or feel unwanted, we want to feel better. We want to feel loved. That's human nature. Nobody says, "I love being angry with my son. It rocks!" We commiserate with friends, speak to spouses, share with co-workers—we will talk with anyone who will listen—all in the attempt to not be mad at our child.

We are eager to return to the good feelings of love and joy. We're looking for someone to validate our feelings and lovingly say, "Ah, poor baby. It sucks, doesn't it? It's all going to be okay. Here, let me hold you."

And that's what junk food does when you think about it. It "makes it all better." Or so we feel in the moment.

You see how this works?

We don't eat what we know isn't good for us (or too much of what is) because we're hungry. We eat it 'cause we have a feeling we can't or don't want to face.

The bedrock of our "habit"—remember we're talking unconscious and repetitive behavior—is how we use food. If we ate only when we were hungry, responding to what our body told us, we'd be fine. The problem is we've learned to believe food can take away all those hard, unwanted feelings:

- Sadness
- Depression
- Anger
- Guilt
- Shame
- Frustration
- Stress

Eventually, if we don't understand what's going on or if we don't know other ways to handle it, we give in, rip open the bag of chips, and dive head-first into forget-the-pain-land. Sure, we promise ourselves that we'll only "eat a few," but really, whom are we kidding? "A few" becomes, "just a few more."

We tell ourselves we will stop anytime. Ah, but we don't.

Food is comfort. And until we are as "comfortable" as we would be if we were just sitting on the dock of the bay, watching the ships roll in, we aren't gonna stop eating.

Let's Play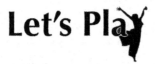

What are your comfort foods?

Remember, we're trying to go from unconscious to conscious. We want to transform our pesky food "habit" into a non...habit. And the only way we're going to be able to see comfort foods for what they are is to take them out for a spin. You don't have to, like, buy them a cute outfit, cruise Van Nuys Boulevard, or introduce them to your boss. But you do have to acknowledge them. Bring them into the light and see them for what they are.

So let's write them down in our journal. Go ahead, let yourself admit it. You swoon at a Hostess Cupcake. You drool around Zebra Popcorn. You go misty eyed at a S'mores Frap from Starbucks. (No, wait—that's Cindy.)

So now write down your foods.

Got them all written?

Good.

Now draw them. Yes. We said draw them. Have fun with this.

You can draw them as the evil little Devil Dogs that they are. Put word bubbles above their rotten little heads and have them say whatever you want them to say.

What the heck. Why don't you draw yourself standing next to them, but not eating them. You are slaying those food dragons.

If you really want to get the full effect, get a towel from the bathroom and safety pin it to your shirt like a cape, then stand up straight and tall (ignoring that nagging backache for just a second) and put your hands on your hips, puff out your chest. (Bonus points for doing all of this in front of a fan; it really adds to the feeling.) Then boldly state, "Be gone, cupcake! You shall never have power over me again!"

Too much?

In that case, ignore the costume but repeat the mantra. (Although we know you really wanted to do the whole megilla.)

Either way, good job. Even without the towel, you're a rockin' super hero. Green Lantern has nothing on you.

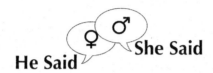

He Said She Said

This time we thought we'd demonstrate what we've learned in screenplay format.

INT – CINDY'S KITCHEN – NIGHT

It's dark. The freezer is wide open and casting a dim light in the room. Cindy is bent over, butt sticking out, deep inside the Kenmore, scarfing up anything that isn't nailed down. There are candy wrappers and cookie dough droplets littered all over the floor like fat confetti. We hear footsteps. Uh-oh. Now Scott's voice –

SCOTT (VO)

Sis? You down there?

Cindy stands, panic stricken. She looks like she's been caught. She slams the freezer shut and frantically starts grabbing up her litter before Scott appears. But she's not fast enough.
Scott enters the room. Sees the litter on the floor, Cindy's face covered in chocolate and marshmallow cream.
SCOTT:

Cindy?

An understanding smile crosses his lips, and he shakes his head. He isn't mad. Or disappointed. He says nothing.

CINDY:

I'm stressed. I'm tired, and I think I should get a job at Costco. I can't write this book.

SCOTT:

(looking at the ice cream container in her hands)

And you thought Ben and Jerry would help?

(Cindy nods.)

CINDY:

It's Phish Food—

Scott looks at the litter of food. He shakes his head.

SCOTT:

And everything else in the fridge—

Cindy looks at the mess on the floor. The junk in her hands—

CINDY:

It's gonna take me a month of walking to make up for this. I can't walk that much. I have deadlines—

Cindy opens the freezer and grabs the first thing she sees. It's a bag of frozen Tater Tots. She rips them open. And pulls one out. Ah, hell, she'll eat it frozen.
Scott walks up to her. He gently takes the Tots from her hands and puts them back where they belong. He closes the freezer.

SCOTT:

Ah, poor baby. It sucks, doesn't it? It's all going to be okay. Here, come here—

He opens his arms for a hug. She accepts.

SCOTT:

Ready to go back to work?

She nods. Cindy returns to life comforted by her brother's hug.

CHAPTER 4: WHY POSITIVE SELF-TALK MATTERS

The World According to Sc⊕tt

The siren call of fame and fortune beckon from Southern California. I am convinced that a Hollywood mogul soon will bathe me in riches and adulation to serve as executive producer of my new reality TV series targeted at those of us forever fighting a growing midsection. "Love ya, baby. Have your people call mine, and we'll do lunch. Well, maybe we'll do salad."

The theme? "Outgrow – Outweigh – Outwit."

Here's the treatment. We all know that the more time pants hang in the far reaches of the closet, the increased likelihood they will be too small when we try them on at a later date. Those extra few nibbles from our kid's plate, grocery store samples, and late night snacks are completely unrelated to our trousers' increased tightness. Therefore, it stands to reason that not wearing an article of clothing over a long period makes it shrink. Examine the garment label; I'm sure it's in the fine print.

So, work with me here. Based on that concept, I see a human drama occurring each morning while the internal debate of what to wear rages. Instead of eating bugs or jumping from buildings—with heart pounding in our ears—we enter the most fearsome part of the closet: that dark, dank, dusty section where outfits we will "get back into one of these days" hang sadly forgotten. Using jumpy, grainy, hand-held, cinema-verité techniques, our POV is a plentiful plethora of peacoats and paisley pants. Tension escalates and drums pound as the contestant must wear the very first pair of slacks he touches! Excuses are barred; explanations such as "last night's dinner was a special celebration" carry no water with the waistline referee. One will be voted out of the closet for comments such as, "I'll wait until I lose a few pounds before I try this one" or "That's odd. They fit last week."

With any challenge, there must be rules. Holding in your stomach to tighten the belt: acceptable. Lying on the bed to fasten the zipper: you're fired!

Oh, wait, I haven't even told you about the part where they eat the disgusting foods. How about lettuce without salad dressing, for a starter?

Words have impact

So we all agree that we're not this size because we eat only when we're hungry. We are this size because we eat to assuage our feelings. But that still doesn't explain why we eat *so* much of the food that's bad for us.

The problem is what we tell ourselves while we're eating those comfort foods.

Do you get that? Let us repeat it. It's important.

The problem isn't that we're eating those foods. It's what we say to ourselves *while* we're eating them. It's those pesky little voices between our ears.

Words are über powerful. Kingdoms are gained and lost on a word. Two words: "I do." Yet think of all the history and life those two little words entail. And "War!" Wow. That's a word isn't it? One little three-letter word. What happens when someone shouts that?

(Or "food fight" in a high school cafeteria. Remember the mayhem—and hoopla—that caused?)

You see. Words really can topple empires. Imagine what they can do to little old us? Think about it—the reason it's illegal to throw insults at children (and why we don't scream insults to others) is because words are powerful. And when our self-talk becomes nothing but a diatribe of vitriol, picture what it can do:

It's evening, and Betty Boomer and her husband Bob have had a tough day. Why? (You fill in the blanks this time. Is it tough co-workers? Waiting on a blood test? A sick sister?)

And on top of that, Betty Boomer and her hub-ster, Bob, are tired. Thinking is the last thing they want to do. They just want to sit down and watch *Star Trek* reruns. (*Next Gen*—not the original *Star Trek*—although we are aware that some might disagree with us, we think Picard is a god.)

Anyway, it's the long end of a very hard day. Bob and Betts are on the couch watching TV, and they are having trouble concentrating on the show 'cause they have so many feels roiling around. What do they do? What do they do?

Do they turn to each other and say, "Let's turn off the TV and talk about how frustrated I am"? No! They don't want to burden their respective spouses. Betty and Bob care for each other; they want to enjoy each other's company. And they don't want to go "there," because "there" is icky and hard, and they want to have fun. Except those sour feelings won't go away. They sit in their guts like thirty-year-old Scooter Pies.

But they need to do something to feel better, so... Betty gets up and dishes out a scoop of mint chip ice cream for herself and another for her hubby.

So now our couple is eating their mint chip on the couch, watching the show. But they aren't paying attention to the ice cream because they can't let go of those pesky feelings. Before they know it, the bowl is empty. And their feelings of frustration have come rushing back.

However, now they are not merely frustrated about their jobs; they are angry with themselves for not enjoying the ice cream and for eating the calories in the first place.

And so the inner dialogue begins. Not with each other, but within themselves.

Betty's goes something like this: "You shouldn't have had that ice cream. Fruit would have been better. But you wanted the ice cream. You never get what you want. Why shouldn't you have the ice cream? You deserve a treat. Yeah, well, that treat means you're gonna have to get up an hour earlier to walk. You don't have time to get up an hour earlier. You've got to take the dog to the vet. Urgh. Why did you eat that ice cream? You could have had half as much. Idiot! You are so dumb. You knew better..."

Poor Betty. What should have been a lovely little treat has now crossed over into a pile of awful, because she's heaped guilt on top of eating the ice cream on top of frustration at work. Too tired and overwhelmed to deal with her "failure," she decides she will diet tomorrow when she feels better, saying "I blew it. Well, as long as I blew it, I might as well really blow it!"

Rationalization firmly in place, the scoops of ice cream give way to a pound of chips, a package of sliced cheese, a box of Lucky Charms, twenty-three pretzel rods, and a loaf of soft, doughy sourdough slathered with warm butter.

So we can clearly see that what started as a means of trying to feel better—a simple scoop (albeit a large one) of Häagen Dazs has horribly backfired. And it was all because of the words Betty told herself.

Since we think in words, and since our thoughts help generate our feelings, what we say to ourselves matters far more than we realize, especially when it has to do with what we weigh. We are just so invested in that number on the scale.

WHY DO WE LIVE AND DIE BY THE SCALE?

We tie our self-worth to the number on the scale. When those numbers head downward, we feel good about ourselves. Should the trend be reversed, so is our mood.

There are probably a million-plus reasons why we value that number on the scale: We were taught to, society tells us to, our doctor warns us to. But that's not what counts here. What matters is that too much food translates into weight gain. Period. End of story. And the next time we weigh ourselves, and the scale's LED confirms the worst, even though we knew it was coming, it still feels like crap. Our internal dialog ramps up, and it's anything but complimentary.

And because we're saying all these terrible things to ourselves, we want to feel better. And since comfort food has always been there, and we don't have to think about it, we have just one bite. But we're "dieting" so we feel bad about that one bite. And so we tell ourselves we're failures, and we feel bad that we're failures, so we have another bite, and that makes us feel bad about ourselves, and so we have another bite. It's *Quantum Leap,* and we're Scott Bakula. Each time we think we're done, we're sucked back in with no Dean Stockwell to guide us.

See how we've come full circle?

Our feelings triggered excessive eating, which caused us to feel bad about ourselves, which caused us to need comfort, which caused us to eat more…and on it goes.

THE CYCLE LOOKS LIKE THIS:

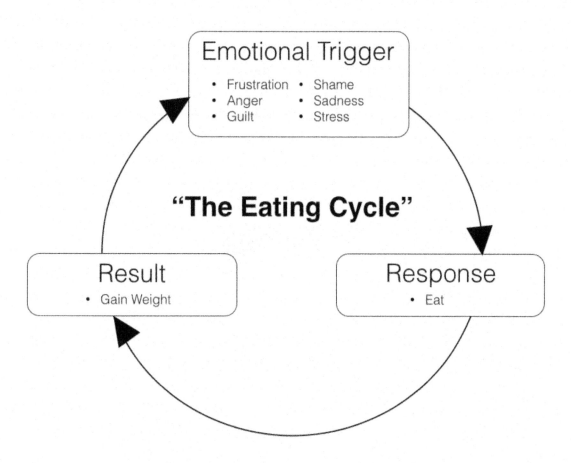

Let's look at the three legs in the cycle:
- Emotional Trigger leads to Eating
- Eating leads to Weight Gain
- Weight Gain leads to Emotional Trigger

We need to understand that we cannot change leg number two because it's simply a reflection of how many calories we took in versus how many we expended. When we eat a lot, we take in more calories than we put back out. It's math (it sucks, but it's math); calories in versus calories out; and no amount of wishin' and hopin' and thinkin' and prayin' and plannin' and dreamin' can undo it. Therefore, once it occurs, weight gain is inevitable. It's gonna happen, and there's not a gosh durn thing we can do about it.

But that still leaves two opportunities to break the cycle. Two opportunities! That's two out of three chances to turn the cycle around. Those are better than Vegas odds!

Go us!

Let's Play
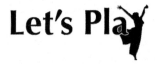

This will be fun!

Get out your notebook.

Now write down ten things you did today that you liked. (If you're really getting into it, list eleven. Aw, what the heck, go hog wild—um, no pun intended—and write down fifteen if you want!) They can be anything. *Anything*! Here are a few suggestions: You were nice to the dog. You smiled at an old woman walking down the street. Your boss said you rocked. You had salad instead of fries for lunch. You didn't leave the kitchen a mess when you went to bed. You brushed your teeth.

If you like, you can underline each thing in a different color. Maybe put a sticker by each item? That's up to you.

But do write at least ten.

Now here comes the hard part:

Write something you like about you. Just one thing you like about who you are We have found, working with the many, many, many people we coach, that this is the hardest exercise of all. Asking people to say one thing they like about themselves. It brings many to tears 'cause they can't find anything. If that's the case for you—and we hope it isn't—here are a few things *we* like about you—

1.   You are smart. You know a lot about eating.

2.   You care. A lot. Isn't that why you need comfort foods? 'Cause your friends and family matter, and you don't want anyone to be sad or in pain?

3.   Maybe the coolest thing is that you bought this book, which means you care about yourself, and you like us! (That means we really like you. As a matter of fact, don't tell the other readers, but you're our favorite reader of all of them. Shhh! Keep it under wraps, okay? If they know that you are our favorite, they'll feel bad about themselves, wondering why they're inadequate. Then, they'll go eat to make themselves feel better. They'll gain weight. They'll tell everyone it was because of this book. Our sales will plummet. Our publisher will drop us. We'll go broke. We'll eat to deal with the fear of becoming homeless, which means we'll gain our weight back. Our reputations will be ruined, and we'll never write another book, instead ending up running a secondhand seventies retro store in Sidney, Nebraska—um, nothing against Sidney Nebraska. We're sure it's a fine place. Anyway? There's a lot riding on your silence, so don't break foul on us, please. Hmmm, maybe we shouldn't have told you in the first place. Oh well

Great job! You are totally bitchin'. And now that you have these things written down, don't stop there. Every day for the next week, before you go to sleep, write down ten things you did that you liked. And if you can, write one new thing each day that you liked about yourself.

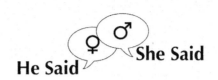

He Said — She Said

We thought it would be fun to make this a music video—sort of. Well, it's a compilation of song lyrics from our youth that tells a story...about a girl, and a boy and a...celebration.

So imagine it. Cindy and Scott dressed in their Baby Boomer duds. Remember those? Bellbottoms. Powder blue leisure suit. Gold chains. (Heaven help us) platform shoes. Love beads. Cindy has long, straight hair ('cause this is a fantasy sequence, and Cindy never in her entire life had long, straight hair—this is her moment!). Scott has those mutton-chop sideburns. (We're really sorry that you will have to scrub these images from your brain later, but we needed to set the full scene. Please forgive us.)

And, honestly, we look like idiots, but hey, we're total rock stars, so we can totally get away with this. We're that bitchin'. Oh yes, we are!

So break out your air guitar and see if you can remember these golden oldies. Oh, oh, and—no cheating by peeking ahead, but at the end of this section we have included the artists who made these great songs famous. See if you can guess them first, before you read the answers. And bonus points if you know the songwriter. But (sad face) there's no prize. Only bragging rights at your next gathering.)

CINDY:

Hey, hot stuff. Are the boys back in town?

SCOTT:

At the Y.M.C.A.

CINDY:

Well, it's another Saturday night. And I just want to celebrate! (Cindy beams, showing off her gams.) Hot legs.

SCOTT:

Bicycle race?

CINDY:

Happy days.

SCOTT:

Let's get down tonight. Boogie. Oogie. Oogie.

CINDY:

Wait! I left my cake out in the rain—

SCOTT:

MacArthur Park?

(Cindy nods)

SCOTT:

Ain't that a shame.

CINDY:

Yeah, cause I'll never have that recipe again.

SCOTT:

Well, you can't always get what you want—

CINDY:

You took the words right out of my mouth.

SCOTT:

Wanna go downtown?

CINDY:

And dance the night away?

SCOTT:

We'll grab the big yellow taxi.

CINDY:

Money?

SCOTT:

A deuce.

CINDY:

Then, we'll take the long way home.

SCOTT:

(pointing to the door) Show me the way.

CINDY:

Follow me, follow you.

(Cindy and Scott head to the door. Scott looks at Cindy. There's a light in his eyes that could give the sun a run for its money. He gets that sweet, loving face that says, "I love you, Sis," but says,)

SCOTT:

Hey. Lady. You make my dreams come true.

CINDY:

(Cindy smiles shyly. She gets all teary) Aw, Bro, I'm a believer.

SCOTT:

Come on. You should be dancin'.

(And the brother-and-sister team head out into the night to celebrate what they have done, giving each other words of encouragement and support 'cause they know kind words generate good feelings, which lead to successful weight control.)

Spoiler Alert! Spoiler Alert! Here be the answers to the Song Title Quiz.
Give yourself a point for every song you got right and the artist who made it popular. Yes, some of these songs are covers. We know that. Some of the artists were popular in our house, and maybe you loved a different version. That could be a total bummer for you. But as Guido says, "Hey, we make-a da game, so we make-a da rules."
1."Hot Stuff," sung by Donna Summer, written by: Pete Bellotte, Harold Faltermeyer, Keith Forsey
2."The Boys are Back in Town," sung by Thin Lizzy, written by Phil Lynett
3."Y.M.C.A.," sung by the Village People (young man) and written by Jacques Morali and Victor Willis (young man)

4. "Another Saturday Night," sung by Cat Stevens. (If you're an audiophile you know that Sam Cooke also made this song famous, 'cause he actually wrote this song. So, if you insist, you can have a point if you said the song was made famous by Sam.)

5. "I Just Want to Celebrate," sung by Rare Earth, written by Dino Fekaris and Nick Zesses

6. "Hot Legs," sung by Rod Stewart, written by Stewart and Gary Grainger

7. "Bicycle Race," sung by Queen (the champions, my friend) and written by Freddie Mercury.

8. "Happy Days" (theme song), sung by Jim Haas and written by Norman Gimble and Charles Fox.

9. "Get Down Tonight," sung by KC and the Sunshine Band, written by Harry Wayne Casey and Richard Finch.

10. "Boogie oogie oogie", sung by Taste of Honey and written by (yes, this song was actually written by someone) Fonce and Larry Mizell.

11. "MacArthur Park," sung by Donna Summer (yes, it was also made famous by Richard Harris, but we like the Donna Summer version, so you can have half a point if you said Richard Harris—how's that?). The song was written by Jimmy Webb.

12. "Ain't That a Shame," sung by Fats Domino, written by Fats and Dave Bartholomew

13. "You Can't Always Get What You Want," sung by the Rolling Stones, written by Mick Jagger and Keith Richards

14. "You Took the Words Right Out of My Mouth," sung by Meat Loaf (Cindy's husband's favorite) and written by Jim Steinman

15. "Downtown," sung by Petula Clark and written by Tony Hatch

16. "Dance the Night Away," sung by Van Halen, written by: Alex, Michael, and Eddie Van Halen, and David Lee Roth

17. "Big Yellow Taxi," sung by Joni Mitchell and written by Joni

18. "Money," sung by Pink Floyd, written by Roger Waters

19. "Deuce," sung by Kiss, written (on a bus) by Gene Simmons

20. "Take the Long Way Home," sung by Super Tramp and writen by Rick Davies and Roger Hodgson
21. "Show Me the Way," sung by Peter Frampton, written by Frampton
22. "Follow Me, Follow You," sung by Genesis, written by: Tony Banks, Phil Collins (huh, who knew?) and Mike Rutherford
23. "Lady," sung by Lionel Ritchie and written by Kenny Rogers.
24. "You Make My Dreams Come True," sung by Hall and Oates, written by Hall, Oates, and Sara Allen.
25. "I'm a Believer," sung by the Monkees, written by Neil Diamond.
26. "You Should be Dancing," sung by the Bee Gees, and written by Barry, Robin and Maurice Gibb

So, how many tunes did you know? And were you able to name the singers? What about the song writers? Groovy you!

If you got 55 points or more, that means you knew the songs and the artists, and you are a god among men (or women). A righteous dude. You shall live long and prosper. And totally deserve to take a bow. (Go on now. Stand up, place one hand in front of your waist, one behind your back, and bow. Hear the thunderous applause (Yay! Clap, clap, clap)…and then get out of the house, 'cause really, you are spending way too much time at home playing Trivial Pursuit.)

If you got 40 to 54 points you are a Bitchin' Bad Ass.

If you got 29 to 39 points you are Gnarly Know It All.

If you got 19 to 28 points you are Rockin' Rock Star.

If you got 18 or fewer points? Bummer, dude. *(Maybe you should go hang out with the chick who got all fifty- five points? Take her to a club. Listen to some music…. She really needs to get out of the house.)*

You do rock. And what you tell—or sing—to yourself matters. So say something nice to you! We know you want to keep the sing-along going, and hey, you play a pretty mean air guitar, but put it away for the moment and tell yourself something complimentary *now*. The air guitar—and that drum set down in the basement that you've turned your mind's eye to—will still be there when you're finished.

CHAPTER 5: FROM WHY TO HOW

The World According to Sc🌐tt

Today, dear traveler, we shall venture into the land of the salad bar, a glorious and wondrous place for dieters. Please keep hands and arms away from the sneeze guard at all time.

There are two types of bars: one consists of leafy lettuce, crinkle-cut carrots, and sliced celery, nested in clear glass bowls. These veggies frustratingly swirl about in craters of ice, making it impossible to use the supplied (always incorrect) utensil to retrieve anything. Periodically, baby corn or garbanzo beans add some taste to this bland assortment of fibrous, flavorless, foods. Since such a salad bar is indeed simply a "salad bar," there is no reason to maximize intake. Just grab a small plate and move on.

We now venture into the holy land of the deluxe salad bar. Look at all those olives (green and black), pickles, pasta salad, macaroni salad, potato salad, and carrot salad. This hodgepodge of sub-salads is reason enough to rejoice, yet the rumbling joy in one's belly is merely beginning.

We leave the concept of "salad" in our wake as we can load our plate with thick fried potatoes, tater rounds, French fries, and mashed potatoes. A multi-cultural experience commences as fried chicken, mini-tacos, pizza, and egg rolls share space with sushi, tempura, and spaghetti, leaving just enough room for a bowl of cheddar cheese, cream of potato, or taco soup.

While steadying precariously this collected cornucopia of caloric courses, add crackers (Saltine or breadstick), bread, rolls, and a bagel, each slathered with butter, cream cheese, or peanut butter. Hang from the thumb, the wire tray compilation of aluminum tins holding a treasure trove of flavored jams, jellies, and preserves.

With experience, one can further learn to balance chocolate, vanilla—or the more exotic tapioca pudding. A second bowl allows for a choice of three flavors of ice cream, chocolate syrup, maraschino cherries, and, of course, whipped cream.

One might wonder why I have strayed from discussing salad dressings. (You'll find them next to the impulse items: bacon bits, croutons, sunflower seeds, raisins, peanuts, and crispy fried noodles.) The answer? It would be wrong; after all, one chooses salad bars to watch one's weight.

And now a brief word from our sponsor...

"Hi, I'm Habit. So, like—'hi.' Yeesh, you've been hearing a lot about me in this book, and you're going to hear a heck of a lot more about me before we're done. You might be asking yourself,, 'Hey, Self, why do they keep going on and on and on about habit? Crikey. I get it. Habits are bad. I've got to drop them.' Yep, you might indeed be saying that.

"However, no offense intended, you'd be wrong. You see, habits, that's me —"hi"—are not necessarily bad. I simply *am*. Period. Actually, I was created to help you. If you think about it, your life is built on me. I kinda rock. I make it easier for you to get everything done and to survive.

"Think of your typical day. Each time there's me, a habit – "hi", I'm going to ding a bell. (It's kind of Pavlovian, so if you're going to drool, please cover the book.) Most likely you get up at the exact same time right down to the minute. (Ding!) You have a morning pattern that consists of a shower (Ding!)—or not (Ding!)—and your standard bathroom rituals. (Ding!) (Ding!) (Ding!) You're either a breakfast eater or you're not. (Ding!) (Ding!) If you are, did you know that there are over 70,000 foods in a standard grocery store? And if you eat breakfast, you probably eat from the same half dozen choices over and over again, (Ding!) prepared in the same fashion you always prepare them. (Ding!) Your daytime pattern is consistent. If you're retired, you fall into a pattern of doing the same things over and over. (Ding!) (Ding!) (Nap.) (Ding!) If you're still "taking what they're giving 'cause you're working for a living," you leave for the job at the same time (Ding!), drive the same roads (Ding!), or take the same bus, train, or subway (Ding!) (Ding!) or (Ding!), arrive at the same time (Ding!), greet the same people (Ding!) (Ding!) (Ding!) (Ding!) (Ding!), have the same conversations (Ding!) (Ding!) (no one talks to Harriet; she's so catty) (Ding!), go to the same restaurants (Ding!)—or bring the same lunches—(Ding!), leave at the same time

(Ding!), drive the same path home (Ding!) (Honk! Honk!) (Ding!), or take the same bus, train, or subway (Ding!) (Ding!) or (Ding!), which is late as usual (Ding!), eat dinner at the same time as always (Ding!) from the same dozen foods (Ding!) (Ding!) (Ding!), watch the same TV shows (Ding!) (Ding!) or read the same authors if you're not a TV person (Ding!) (Ding!), collapse into the same chair or the same place on the couch (Ding!), go to bed at the same time (yawn, Ding!)—and most likely sleep with the same person every night (Ding!) (Hubba hubba!) (Ding!)

Habit. (Ding!) Habit. (Ding!) Habit. (Ding!)"

Now, I'm not pointing this out to make you think you're living in that first Apple MacIntosh commercial, the one that looked like *1984*. (What did that commercial mean anyway? And did you know it aired only one time? Really. Throw that in your trivia game question hopper.)

It's just, picture the alternative, waking up every single day with *no* routines. No me, Habit – "hi!" - At first, you'd feel like you were on an extended vacation, exciting and new, welcome aboard. But after a while, your head would start spinning. As Jack Nicholson kinda sorta said to Tom Cruise, "You need habits on that wall!" Without me, habit – "hi" , you would get exhausted. So you see, I, Habit – "hi!" – can be pretty cool. So that's, it. Thanks for listening. This is Habit, signing off. "Goodnight and—"Bye."

We now return to our regularly scheduled book...

Heed this *(ominous music please):* When the pain of the habit's side effect becomes more damaging than the benefit of the habit's intent, it's time to change the habit.

Read that line over again. It's possibly the most important line in this book.

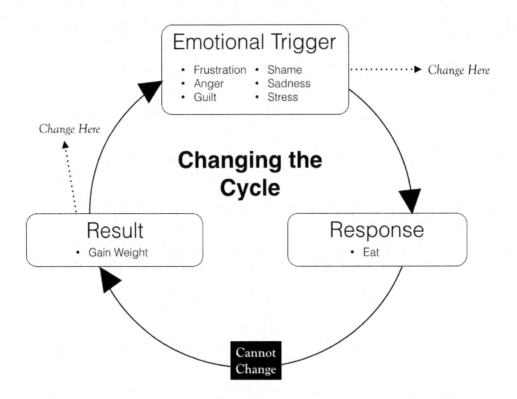

Habitual eating—or the unconscious eating that makes us put on weight—begins with an emotional reaction. The emotion is one that that we don't want, like anger or frustration or even boredom. It can be something going on right now, or even something from our past (like those ugly gym clothes you used to have to wear for P.E. Really? Being an adolescent wasn't tough enough without having to wear those? Gag me with a spoon.) To make the feeling go away, we seek comfort. Since we associate comfort with food—we eat. We know eating for the wrong reasons is only going to send our efforts down the tubes, but there we are doin' it anyway. We berate ourselves for being weak and giving in, which makes us feel worse and makes us need more comfort, which means we eat more, which makes us berate ourselves for eating, so we want more comfort, etc....

So how do we stop the cycle? We have two options.

Option 1: Change your internal dialogue

__Old scene__:

You're standing on the scale, and you see you have a two-pound gain. "That's bogus," you say, "That can't be right."

You remove your shoes, your belt, your watch—you even try exhaling hard, trying to remove anything from your person that could possibly cause the scale to go up like that. You weigh yourself again, this time trying all sort of different positions (which we call "scale surfing"), trying to get the number to change.

No luck. You're still up two pounds. *"Two pounds!"* you yell. "This is so unfair!"

In rushes the gamut of emotions. They range from crummy to crummier.

(Since you know *Old scene* all too well, we won't go into details here of what you do when those crummy feelings arise. After all, if we get too detailed, you'll feel bad, forget about reading the remainder of this book, and attack the peanut butter.)

__New scene__:

You get on the scale and it's the exact same situation—but let's make one *minor* adjustment:

This two-pound gain is *after* you just returned from a two-week all-expense paid luxury cruise on The Love Boat.

Well, Dyn-o-mite! You're pleased as sugar-free Kool Aid, possibly even ecstatic, because you put on *only* two pounds. A luxury cruise like that, with Gopher and Captain Stubing—you should have put on a good 7 to 10 pounds.

Now, instead of hiding from the gain, you're calling your friends: "Dude! You won't believe this! You know that cruise we just took, the one with twenty-four-hour all-you-can eat buffet? Guess what, I only gained two pounds!" This is more fun than playing in refrigerator boxes or building living room forts. Yes sir-ee, Bob! You are indeed one foxy mama.

When you look at it honestly, both are identical, right?

In each case you're now tipping the scale at 32 more ounces than you did the last time you checked—it's 2 pounds either way.

The only thing that's different is the words you told yourself.

In *Old scene* you punished yourself and were generally unkind to you. You beat yourself up for being a failure. You were singing "Eve of Destruction." With your self-esteem shot to hell, of course you gave up trying. Who wouldn't?

In *New scene*, Edwin Hawkins and his singers are backing you up with "Oh, Happy Day!" But really, you simply placed your weight gain in perspective and told yourself kind things. You celebrated what you were able to do, and your self-esteem went up. You felt empowered.

And the more empowered you feel, the less your need to artificially comfort yourself. With that trigger unpulled, you make healthier choices, which further empowers you.

That's so important that we are going to say it again. (Insert sound of cassette tape rewinding while you're holding down the Play button at the same time.) **The more empowered you feel, the less your need to artificially comfort yourself. The result is you will make healthier choices, which further empowers you.**

Stated yet one more way: When you cut yourself some slack, instead of finding yet another reason to beat yourself up, you lessen the compulsion to "eat away" the feelings. That, in turn, helps you stick with your program, hopefully letting you drop a few pounds, further amplifying positive feelings, encouraging more success. Dig?

The bottom line is: If you want to permanently change what you weigh, change what you say, which is a cool mantra to put on your refrigerator. "If you want to change what you weigh, change what you say." This alters the entire cycle, helping to ensure success. Plus, let's be honest, isn't it a lot more fun to wake up each day feeling good about yourself?

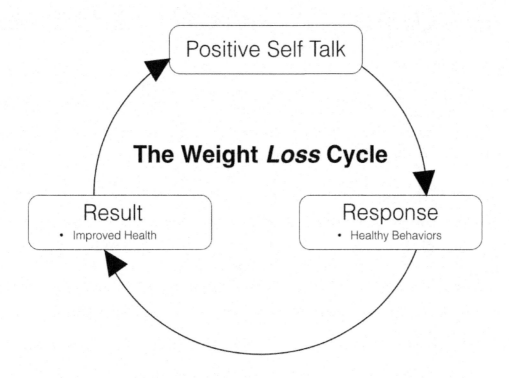

The Weight *Loss* Cycle

- Positive Self Talk
- Response
  - Healthy Behaviors
- Result
  - Improved Health

Option 2: Change what you do

No emotion, no matter how happy or sad, *makes* us eat. Eating as a reaction is something we have learned over time. But since we have learned this reaction, we can also unlearn it!

That's important so let's repeat it. In fact, say it aloud:

"What I have learned I can unlearn. I'm that powerful!"

HOW DO WE UNLEARN UNHEALTHY EATING?

1. Understand unhealthy eating is tied to your emotions.

2. Stop "white knuckling."

"White knuckling" is trying to *push* your way through a habit change. White knucklers stand around with their hands balled into fists and repeat the mantra: "I will not eat. I will not eat. I will not eat." White knucklers can indeed avoid unhealthy eating with this very difficult technique; however, the entire time they're saying "I will not eat," they are focusing front and center, tooth and nail, hither and yon, on the very thing they want to do: eat.

White knuckling won't work. It can't. And it's too hard. Besides, it's not a fun way to live life. And it gives you hand cramps, and it makes your skin look older (which it's already doing way too quickly anyway). And let's be real, what usually happens, in the end, is that white knucklers get so stressed out from focusing on what they can't do, they say, "Ah screw it, I'll just do it this one time." They give in. Cue flood gates opening.

HOW DO YOU NOT "WHITE KNUCKLE?"

First, you need to identify your trigger.

A trigger is an emotion that's highly charged. For some people their trigger is sadness. When they are sad, they are triggered to eat. Does that make sense? For some their trigger is anger. When they are angry, they are triggered to eat. Many of us have more than one trigger.

Here are just a few of the triggers we've faced:

1. Sadness.
2. Anger
3. Stress
4. Confusion
5. Boredom
6. Depression
7. Anxiety

There are a lot of them. And as we said earlier, most of us have more than one trigger.

Now that you know what your trigger is, you need to create a plan.

A plan is exactly like it sounds. It's an action that takes you from the charged eating situation into a new, healthy situation where you won't give in to Mr. Carbalicious.

Here's how it works:

Let's say, one of your triggers is stress (whose isn't?), and you have realized and *now accept* that you are triggered to eat in reaction to stress—and, best of all, you have made the decision to change. You have decided that stress will no longer be a trigger for you; you will no longer eat as a reaction to stress.

Good for you.

Your next step is to come up with a plan because you don't want to white knuckle. Remember, when we fail to plan, we plan to fail. And since stress always has a way of finding us, no matter how we want to avoid it, having a plan to succeed is really, *really* important.

So the next time you feel stressed out, you will take a walk, or you will call a friend, or you might even do something as simple as get out of the room for ten minutes.

Voila! You have created a plan. It's that simple.

Let's Play

Get out your journal.

We're going to practice positive self-talk.

Write down three positive things you can say to yourself should you end up eating inappropriately or when comfort foods take over your brain.

Here are a few things Cindy says to herself:

• *"So I blew it. It's done. You had a crap day. It's okay. You're human. You can start again tomorrow. Or you can start again right now."*

• *"This Hostess Snowball will never taste as good as those size 3 shorts feel!"*

• *"You ate that Hostess Cupcake. That's okay. It was just one. You can still get on top of this. Think about how cute you look in that dress and how it doesn't pull like it used to. You did that. You made it fit like a dream. And you can do this. It's just a lousy cupcake."*

Here are a few things Scott says to himself:

• *"I make mistakes because I am human. Becoming aware of my mistakes gives me the power to correct them.*

• *I treat myself the same way I treat other people I care about when they make mistakes."*

• *"You ate that Hostess Cupcake. Think about how cute you look in that dress and how it doesn't pull like it used to."* (Okay, Scott really wouldn't say this because he doesn't wear dresses—well, at least not that we know of. But certainly not when he's eating cupcakes. We're 99% sure of that.)

Use what we wrote or write something new.

Good job!

He Said   She Said

A phone conversation between Cindy and Scott.
Scott's at home. His phone rings.
BRRRing. BRRRing.
Scott picks it up

SCOTT:

Go for Scott.

CINDY:

Scott?

SCOTT:

Hey you, what's up?

CINDY:

I am so stressed! *I have two scripts due next week!* Finn has a crapload of doctors' appointments, and I can't cancel again or they'll start charging me. Flip's out of town, so he can't take him. We have this new kid staying with us who needs my time. *I really want candy!*

SCOTT:

No. You don't.

CINDY:

Nah huh. You're not the boss of me. *(mumble grumble)* Idotoowantcandy.

SCOTT:

How about a bath? You like baths.

CINDY:

(still mumbling) Bathsarestupid.

SCOTT:

Go put the water on. I'll wait here.

CINDY:

But you're busy—

SCOTT:

Yes, but you matter to me...
Cindy gets all sniffly.

CINDY:

I do?

Cindy cries and lets out everything that's been bothering her. Scott listens. Her sniffles subside.

SCOTT:

You okay?

CINDY:

Yeah.

SCOTT:

You gonna eat?

CINDY:

No.

SCOTT:

I'm proud of you.

CINDY:

Love you, bro. Thanks.

SCOTT:

Love you too.
(They hang up. Cindy takes her bath.)

You see how much better that was? Cindy's plan was to call her big bro when stress triggered her. She felt better. They got closer. And Scott was able to help Cindy find a new plan, which was to take a bath. If Cindy didn't have a plan locked in, she would probably still be eating.

CHAPTER 6: HOW DO I CREATE A PLAN?

The World According to Sc🌐tt

A man – a plan – a hanker-an

Yup. A man's gotta do what a man's gotta do.

And right now, after months of lightweight food with no taste—and even less heft—I've got a heavy hankerin' for a triple-meatball, pepperoni sausage, six-cheese submarine sandwich, oozing over a warm, doughy, foot-long toasted Mozzarella Parmesan Italian roll, followed by a family-size order of cottage fries (sans family) smothered in chili cheese sauce. The chaser for this gloriously caloric feast will be a chocolate chunk, hyper-sized milkshake stuffed with peanut butter blobs and overflowing with rich syrup.

I suck in my gut, march boldly into the sandwich shop, and swagger to the counter. Feet planted, I stand my ground in an oh-so-macho fashion and make direct eye contact with the young woman behind the register. Actually, I don't know if young women consider middle-aged, slightly soft, bespectacled, grey-haired men to be manly, but red meat, elevated-cholesterol, saturated-fat meals seem to me a masculine food. I must place myself in the right frame of mind prior to ordering.

She asks, "What would you like?" (I am amazed she is not swooning from the animal magnetism I exude.)

"Forget the calories, Scott. Go for it!" I hear in my head.

Clearing my throat, I deepen my voice, and—for causes unbeknownst to me—reply in a crackling, tinny, scratchy sound, "Veggie sandwich. Diet soda."

Sean Connery had entered the restaurant; Woody Allen had ordered.

~~~

Ah, the best laid plans, huh?

So why do some of our plans succeed? And why do other plans fail—even if they are as simple as ordering a sandwich?

The answer is simple and easy

In order for any plan to work, it must be both simple and easy. If it's simple, but not easy, you won't do it. If it's easy but not simple, it will require too much effort.

Let's say you're going through your closet, trying to find something that fits, and you find your 1970 polyester blend maroon tunic and beige platform shoes, and it brings back so many good memories that you want to re-create them. In a Long Island Iced Tea-induced state of mind, you decide that the very best way to do that would be to become the world's best Baby Boomer hula-hooper. (*This, like so many other ideas we've seen, falls under the category of "It seemed like a good idea at the time."*)

To accomplish this feat, a simple twelve-step plan might look like this:

1.   First of all, sober up. After all, in your state of advanced years you don't want to hula drunk. (*Actually, we don't recommend you hula-hooping to begin with, but if you want to look like a doofus with a cheap, round tube of brightly colored plastic spinning around your bulging midsection, who are we to say you're wrong?*

2.   Go to the store and buy a hula hoop.

3.   Find a large space where you have enough room to wobble, wiggle, and waggle like a post-middle-aged Weeble. (*For everyone's sake, please make it where no one can see you. Jeeze.*)

4.   Place the ring around your hips. (*We're warning you, this won't end well. You can stop now. Really, we're just thinking of you. We've come so far together, we don't want to lose you before you finish our book.*)

5.   Swivel like a 45 rpm record without an adapter spinning on a turntable. (*We can't look. We know what's going to happen.*)

6.   Watch the hoop fall to the ground after, oh, let's say one spin.

7.   Reach down to pick it up, determined to pursue this ridiculous dream. (*For God's sake, we're begging here. Don't do it!*)

8.   Throw your back out while bending over. *(Damn! We knew it. Didn't we warn you? But oh, no, you knew more than us. You had to be a bigshot, didn't you?)*

9.   Drop to the floor writhing in agony, swearing profusely, and calling the hoop a torture device.

10.   Lie on the floor until someone can come home and help you to your bed where—if you're lucky—you will remain for only the next seventy-two hours

11.   Have a family member fetch your laptop once you're able to sit upright so you can send us an e-mail telling us we were right in the first place and you don't know what came over you. *(Don't worry; you're forgiven. But, next time you'll listen, won't you?)*

See? It's very *simple*. We can lay out the steps in a clear, linear fashion that anyone can understand.

The problem is that plan was not *easy*. It would take mental and physical discipline, commitment, patience, and resources (such as doctors and pain meds). Moreover, it requires you to learn new skills.

Even though the plan is simple, the obstacles diminish the likelihood of achieving the goal.

For us to succeed at losing and keeping off weight, our plan must be both simple and easy.

Except losing weight isn't simple, is it?

Our weight is such an emotionally charged issue that we blow our success—and failure—way out of proportion. Our weight loss has more baggage than a Samsonite factory.

Let's explain:

Here is a normal problem, but one we hope you don't really have:

Your roof leaks.

Here is your simple plan to fix it:

1) You admit that there is a leak

2) You identify where the leak is.

3) You seek out a roofer

4) You check the roofer's references

5) You meet with the roofer, agree to a schedule and a fee

6) You and the nice, reputable roofer sign a contract

7) You pay the roofer upon satisfactory completion

See there's no drama or hoopla or angst. You saw the problem with the roof. You fixed it. You didn't berate the issue or struggle with whether it existed or not. You had a problem—your roof leaked—you created a plan, and you implemented it. Done and done.

Ah, but that's not what happens when you decide you have to lose weight, is it? Think about it. If you were to solve the roofing problem the same way you go about losing weight it would look like this:

1) Deny that there's a leak, rationalizing that the look of pots and pans collecting water on the floor is a preferred interior design.

2) After *finally* admitting there is a leak, you indignantly blame the rain, sun, and roof for causing the leak, justifying inaction by saying, "It's not fair and it's not my fault. Why should *I* have to fix it?"

3) You might invite guests to a themed "umbrella party" where you would acknowledge that although there is a leak, and you could fix it anytime, it's not really a problem, so you'll get to it "when the holidays are over."

4) With your furniture mildewed, you would search the internet for "Get Dry Quick" schemes that proclaim, "Don't change a thing! Just buy this product, and the leak will automatically fix itself. No messy tar. No shingles. No patching!"

5)   After wasting countless dollars on "The Secrets Roofers Don't Want You to Know," you become angry, frustrated, overwhelmed—and, of course, very, very wet.

6)   Until you accept the problem and seek help

Losing and maintaining weight is more emotionally charged than the ending to *Brian's Song*. So "simply" having a "simple" plan to take-off weight, and avoid triggers, isn't going to work. If you want to succeed at weight loss, your plan must also be easy.

Therefore, should you wish to move forward *and achieve your goals,* you must set a very simple course *and* it must be easy enough to fit into your life so that it will not disrupt your entire existence. (That's another one of those "read that again" places.) (So do it!)

One of the biggest reasons goals fail is that people make them too complicated for their lives. They just don't fit.

Let's Play

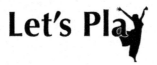

It's time to make a new plan, Stan.

We want to make sure you have your plan thing locked in. We want your plan to be so concrete in your mind that facing down a trigger is easy as—well—pie. (Hmmm. Bad metaphor. How 'bout piece of cake? Nope, not working either.)

Get out your journal, and your pen, and your inner Roy Rogers, and identify at least one trigger. If you have more than one trigger—like us—identify those too.

Now devise a specific plan for you to take when each specific trigger kicks in.

Write down each trigger and each plan in your journal.

Here are a few ideas for plans:

- "When I feel overloaded and inclined to eat, I will go take a bath."
- "During family get-togethers, I will position myself away from the food so I won't be tempted to eat."
- "Instead of eating late at night, I will call a friend." (Of course, it had better be an insomniac friend, or it would be rude. And then you'd feel guilty. And then you'd want to eat, and that would ruin the whole thing.)

That was fun.

Now draw yourself doing your plan.

If your plan is to take a bubblebath when you're sad, draw yourself in the bath, enjoying the peace and comfort. *(Don't worry, no one will see it but you.)*

We encourage you to take that wonderful plan to the next level:

Go buy some bath salts and that yummy soap you've had your eye on, to encourage you to take that warm bath. Pick up those scented candles. Dig out your old macramé candle hangers Fire up the lava lamp. Close your eyes and see yourself taking a bath when you're feeling sad. Make your plan as sensual and real to you as possible.

The more you embrace your plan in your mind, the easier it will be to do when you need it.

Ta-dah!

Small steps done repeatedly will always generate better results over larger steps done once in a while. It's better to commit to walking a block every day—and really do it—then to swear you'll run a mile and never get around to it. Make it simple enough to fit in your life.

If your weight-loss plan is both simple and easy you will stay in the Success Zone.

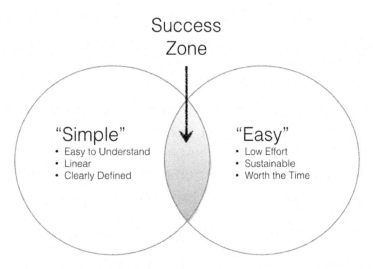

Let's Play

Oh how we love this next game. It's both Simple and Easy which equals fun.

For this game, you are going to need pipe cleaners. You can get them in one solid color, or you can get that fun variety pack with the rainbow assortment. We suggest the longer ones, so your fingers don't get cranky.

Now, we want you to shape the pipe cleaner in the svelte and sexy shape you are now on the road to having. For the gents, give your pipe cleaner dude some beefy muscles, or maybe you want to have a "dad bod" (which we're told by the young'uns, is the body you want to have. Who knew?).

Add as much detail to your pipe cleaner you as you would like. Does your pipe cleaner avatar have hair? What about shoes? Pants? Have fun with this.

Once you have completed this "mini-me" put it where you can see it, as a reminder to keep it simple, easy, and have fun.

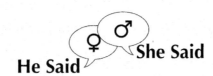

He Said · She Said

For the wrap up, we are going to have a conversation that shows how doing something difficult and complex is simply more work than it's worth.

CINDY:

Oh Scotteth, thou comest upon mine humble abode at a most opportune time, so please come hither, for thou is most needed for the vellum upon which I have extended ink is most in need of your swiftest reply.

SCOTT:

Oh Cindyeth, I am here upon thy beckoning, and I have arrived post haste as thou requested. For what troubles thy brow?

CINDY:

Uncertainty beckons like a darkness in the shadows and fills me with dread for art the words upon this parchment satisfactory?

SCOTT:

You must pulleth thine head thither from thine hindquarters.

CINDY:

Thou areth showing a jerkiness in thy face.

SCOTT:

Closeth thine pie hole.

CINDY:

You closeth thine own pie hole!

Did you get what we were saying?

You see, when something is too difficult and complex, it's just too much work to follow. So keep it simple and easy, and you will have success.

CHAPTER 7: HOW DO WE MAKE OUR DIET "SIMPLE" AND "EASY?"

The World According to Sc🌐tt

Offering up the rationale that she had to go out of town, my trainer canceled our appointment. I knew the *real* reason: She had grown tired of me, leaving to find another greybeard to tutor, tossing me to the curb like yesterday's recyclables. As revenge, I would forgo my exercise regimen, opting instead to sleep late, eat immense amounts of sugary snacks, gain lots of weight, and make her feel guilty. Don't mess with the male ego; it is a bewildering and convoluted place.

However, fate interceded, and my eyes popped open at 3:30 AM, leaving me restless and incapable of returning to the embracing arms of Hypnos. Since I could not sleep, the question became, "What do I do at this hour?"

I could exercise.

The notion of huffing, puffing, bending, and squatting in the cold morning dampness—with no trainer guiding over me and coercing me—struck me as being as appealing as bathing in ice water. Yet, in this pre-dawn mentally fuzzy state, activity sounded more attractive than staring at dark bedroom walls; so I ventured outdoors, thinking, "I can walk to the bakery and get a donut." Strapping on walking shoes, iPod, and fleece vest, I set forth into the inhospitable chilly climes of dawn.

Soon my fitter angels won out; I detoured to the park and was indeed huffing, puffing, bending, and squatting at my usual workout locale. As uncoordinated as I felt, I assumed passing motorists would deduce I was in the midst of a seizure and stop to offer assistance. Since none did, I continued uninterrupted, completing my routine well before the bakery opened. I then urged myself to kill time by actually jogging, establishing short goals to avoid over-exertion.

Upon reaching the sidewalk that bounds the park, I thought, "That's easy," and set my sights for a telephone pole down the block. Pole by pole, house by house, I advanced until, flush with the ecstasy of accomplishment but reaching my limit, I prepared to stop—until I saw a woman running ahead of me.

Still smarting from being jilted by my trainer, a greater cause now made itself known. No longer about my seeking conditioning, this was now a battle between the sexes. For all that is good, noble, and fit in men, I had to outrun this lone female jogger, demonstrating what I could do on my own so I could boast to my trainer, proving my independence.

Summoning all the machismo inherent in a middle-aged, slightly soft, non-runner on the verge of collapse, I nonchalantly accelerated next to her, acting as if this were a typical practice. Without breaking stride, she waved, "Hi."

Attempting to return the salutation with a husky, deep-voiced, "Howdy," I was stunned when, instead of my usual manly, dulcet tones, all that exhaled from 'twixt my lips was a thick, gasping, airy, sickly wheeze, akin to a pipe organ blasting with rotted bellows. Stunned (and probably frightened), her eyes opened huge, and she stopped dead in her tracks.

Humiliated beyond belief, I accelerated with the last remaining tidbits of energy I possessed, disappearing behind a tree and collapsing in the grass, where I lay until I had enough strength to crawl to the bakery and claim my donut.

The KISS principle ("Keep It Simple, Skinny")

It is so easy for our plans to derail, isn't it? And it often feels like sabotage is around every corner. We can feel like Maxwell Smart trying to outmaneuver The Claw. ("It's not the CRAW, it's the CRAW!")

But fear not, brave Boomer, for we have some really great tips that will help you keep your plan on track:

Tip #1: **Tell someone about your plan.**

(We recommend a friend or supportive spouse. We don't advise knocking someone down on the street and forcing them to listen to you. We've found that approach often leads to a cranky and unreceptive listener.) If your friend doesn't have to write down your plan, and can indeed remember it after hearing it once or twice, then give yourself a big KISS, because you've Kept It Simple, Skinny.

Here's an example of a program that Cathy Complicated might try:

1. Weigh and record your weight every day at the same time
2. Exercise for thirty minutes every day
3. Track all foods in a journal (or online)
4. Measure all portions
5. Stay away from fatty foods and sugar
6. Cook in a healthy fashion
7. Eat at least five portions of fruits and vegetables
8. Stop eating by eight o'clock each night
9. Eat at restaurants no more than twice a week
10. Drink six glasses of water every day

And we have to applaud Cathy. So eager to achieve her goals, she has plotted out a very thorough plan. However, what Cathy doesn't realize is:

1. The pursuit of perfection leads to procrastination, which leads to paralysis. Trying to be the "perfect" dieter is actually a barrier to getting most things done. Because Cathy is so busy preparing for each and every possible obstacle, she'll never be able to put her entire plan in motion. In the end, she will end up doing the "When the kids head back to school," denial or the "After the holidays," denial or the "Just this once," denial.

2. Unless she's one of those memory experts who we've seen on shows like *Late Night*, she just won't remember all the nuances to her plan. Easy it is not. And if Cathy has a life, already balancing a pretty active schedule, her weight loss plan will not work, despite all of her good intentions. As they say, "The road to hell is paved with good intentions."

Tip #2: **Use the 80/20 rule**

The 80/20 rule says that 80 percent of all results are generated by 20 percent of all activity. (And yes, it's a real thing. Technically, it's called the "Pareto Principle.") Here's how it works:

Ever been on a committee? Maybe it was at work, at church or synagogue, or when you were involved with your kids' school? And did you ever notice how 80 percent of the work got done by 20 percent of the people? (Most likely, it was you and one or two other people, right?) Anyway, that's the 80/20 rule in day-glo brightness. When there are ten people on a project, two of them will do all the work. (Of course, the others will tell everyone that they did all the work. That's called the "I Always-Take-Credit-for-Everything-Because-I'm-a-Jerk Principle.")

HOW DOES THE 80/20 RULE HELP US LOSE WEIGHT?

The rule tells us is that in actuality, to be successful at weight loss, *all we need to do is devise a plan for the most important 20 percent* of our weight loss issues. Doing that, and that alone, will handle 80 percent of our triggers. And let's be honest, if we lost weight 80 percent of the time, we'd be happy, thin campers, wouldn't we? As a matter of fact, if any part of our life worked out as we wanted 80 percent of the time, we'd be deliriously joyful. (Actually, now that we think about it, there are days we'd take 60 percent. Heck, sometimes 20 seems like a gift.)

So, using Cathy Complicated's example—which had ten items in its plan—she picks the two that are most problematic and focuses on those:

Track and record all foods

Stop eating by eight o'clock each night

Now, with the 80/20 rule firmly in place, and the import of K.I.S.S., Cathy is destined for success.

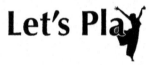

Let's Play

Get out your journal. And your pen.

This is going to be fun because we get to work with columns—four to be exact. So, on your trusty piece of paper make three columns down the length of the page. Here's what ours looks like:

Habit Trigger	Severity of Trigger	How Often?	Score
Late night eating	9	30	☆ 270
Celebrations	10	2	20
Paying bills	7	4	28
Tasting food while cooking	9	40	☆ 360
Going out to eat	6	8	48
Concerns about retirement	10	5	50
Eating at the movies	3	2	6

In Column One—

Write down all the triggers that you can think of that cause you to gain weight. They might include stress, travel, late night eating, being over-worked. List everything!

In Column Two—

Next to each trigger, give it a score. Use 1 to 10, with 10 being a major problem while ONE is only slightly problematic for you.

In Column Three -

Write down how often each event occurs in an average month.

Multiply column two times column three for each item, which will give it a score.

In Column Four –

Beside the item, write your score.

Pick the twenty percent with the highest totals.

Devise a plan to deal with your top twenty percent.

What we want you to notice (aside from the cute stars) is that not all your trigger scores are way up there. In fact, most of your triggers are not as trigger-y as you thought. Do you see how much in control you actually are? Not all your triggers were created equal. That's a lot less overwhelming isn't it?

Ah, but we are not done with this game. We have one more step to go.

We call this step "How to create a plan for the 20 percent" (probably because that's what you're going to do—create a plan to deal with that important 20 percent).

Guess what you get to do?

That's right: Create more columns! Four will do it. Continuing with our example above, we're using the #1 problem we had above, tasting while cooking, and we've listed several techniques we could use.

Possible Solution	How Effective?	How Likely?	Total Score	Rank
1. Never eat again	10	1	10	6
2. Have someone else cook	9	3	27	5
3. Go out to eat	10	5	50	2
4. Chew gum while cooking	8	8	64	1 ☆
5. Listen to music while cooking	3	10	30	4
6. Have pre prepared foods delivered	9	4	36	3

COLUMN ONE

Write down everything you could do to overcome the obstacles you just identified. Don't censor yourself; let your thoughts fly free like butterflies.

COLUMN TWO

Just like you did when you were rating your triggers, rate each action plan on a 1-to-10 basis, with 10 being the most effective as a solution, and 1 being completely ineffective.

And please don't go all logical here. And *be honest!* (Nobody is reading this but you, so yes, it might look cool that you gave jogging a high score.

(But let's be real here. At our age—at least for us (Scott and Cindy)—running just ain't a happening thing. Our flab keeps moving long after we stop. We would, however, love to take Zumba. Or swim. Swimming is a wonderful exercise and makes Cindy really happy. Scott takes Zumba. He even wears those outfits. It's not a pretty picture, but it keeps him fit, so don't judge.)

Write down your *honest* rating for each action you listed.

Multiply column one times column two for each item to get a total.

COLUMN THREE

Write down your score.

Pick the twenty percent with the highest totals; you've probably narrowed it down to two activities, maybe even only one (and in this case you want "one" to be a lonely number). As you can tell, we boiled down all the problems we had into one simple step that will help us lose weight, "Chew gum while cooking."

Do whatever you come up with, starting now! (Well maybe not right now. You may want to finish reading the chapter.)

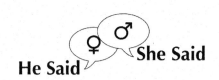

He Said She Said

We thought it would be fun to write this recap with Cindy and Scott in a film noir style.

(A woman steps into the pool of light in the darkened streets of Gotham. We'll call her Cindy – probably because that's her name. She wears a fedora and trench coat and sucks on a lollipop—the Vitamin C kind. Cindy may be noir-y, but she's still healthy. A slutty saxophone plays somewhere in the distance.)

CINDY:

It was a rainy night in Gotham. The streets were emptier than a bag of Pepperidge Farm Cookies at a TOPS convention. I had just closed a case. A farmer. He wanted to know why his chicken had crossed the road. I told 'im, "To get to the other side." "Side of what?" he asked. "What did it matter?" I answered. "East side, west side, all around the town was all the same." We parted ways. And I figured that was it. I was done. The detective game had become too much. A gal couldn't be expected to follow chickens forever. Maybe it was time I threw in the towel. That's when he walked into my life.

(In sashays Scott. He's wearing a floral dress and large Kentucky Derby bonnet. He carries a Hostess Cupcake. Cindy doesn't react to any of it. She doesn't even flinch. She's seen it all.)

SCOTT:

(speaking in a falsetto so high it could curl your hair) You Cindy? The private detective?

CINDY:

Maybe.

SCOTT:

Heard you'll take on the toughest cases.

CINDY:

Maybe I will and maybe I won't.

SCOTT:

No. You gotta help me. You just gotta.

CINDY:

(*to the audience*) I figured the gotta was up for grabs. But there was something in his voice. Something strange. I couldn't put my finger on it. So I said, "What do you need?"

SCOTT:

I need you to listen.

CINDY:

Yeah.

SCOTT:

I'm thinking of losing weight. And I thought if I did Zumba three times a week, instead of one, and drank an extra two glasses of water a day, it would help.

CINDY:

Couldn't hurt.

SCOTT:

You think?

CINDY:

Drink two extra glasses of water and add on two extra classes of Zumba. That's two plus two.

SCOTT:

Yeah. Exactly.

CINDY:

I think you got something there.

SCOTT:

Oh Cindy. Thank you. Can I K.I.S.S. you?

CINDY:

Hey, I ain't that kind of detective.

SCOTT:

I understand. You are who you are.

CINDY:

That's right. I am what I am.

SCOTT:

Still, thanks for the help. You made a huge difference.

CINDY:

All in a night's work.

(Scott sashays off, pleased with his new 80/20 plan.

Cindy smiles. Maybe she won't give up the game. The sax plays on.)

CHAPTER 8: HOW DO I STAY ON TRACK?

The World According to Scott

I have a suggestion for a front-page headline: MARCUS WEARS BELT ONE NOTCH TIGHTER—WITHOUT SUFFOCATING.

I realize there is other news in our little burg nestled on the coast. But—in my world—this headline is a 500-point bold font, above-the-fold, screamer! MY BELT HAS ONE FEWER HOLE TO CONQUER! The public needs to know this. Didn't some philosopher say something akin to, "One man's success enhances everyone?" Therefore isn't it morally wrong to withhold this information from our county?

Okay, I'll admit it's happened before. But on those occasions, I yanked, pulled, and tugged the leather around my midsection to make it stretch, holding in my stomach, not daring to exhale or sit. This time, it's different! I pulled the belt to fasten it, and it went farther—all by itself!

Amazed, I need confirmation in the mirror. Maybe, while I slept, some pod-like aliens substituted for the real me a skinnier version of their human captive. I look. Hmm...grey hair, oversized ears, goatee. Still me. Wow!

I stare intently at my profile in the reflection, pushing in the couple inches around my navel for confirmation. "Houston, we have belt-fastening." I move closer to analyze the image. "By golly, that's definitely my stomach under that taut belt. If this ain't newsworthy, nothing is!"

Since everyone must know, I slide this information into seemingly unrelated conversations.

"Ten dollars," says the store clerk, "Cash or credit card?"

"Credit card," I reply, swaggering and reaching into my back pocket, accentuating my stud-like figure. "You know," I mention casually, "it's much easier to get my wallet now that my belt is tighter." I fix her with a John Wayne stance. She looks at me as if I'm Don Knotts.

I admit I'm proud of this. If I can focus on these little changes in my program, it makes the journey ahead less daunting. So I'll broadcast my success. When I lose 10 pounds, I'm calling *60 Minutes*.

So you're psyched. You've tasted success. Technically we could remove the training wheels from your balloon-tire Schwinn, insert a couple of playing cards in the spokes, attach some streamers to the handlebars, and send you on your merry way, flap-flap-flapping down the road.

Except....

We are Boomers, and we've been around this diet block one too many times. We know that there remain hurdles still out there, lurking in the darkness, like Freddy Krueger—hurdles that, without warning, without mercy, will put an end to our hard-earned glory, pushing us to the fridge, destroying our newly minted success. .

What are these no-good, rotten saboteurs called? They are, *(drama sting, please)* the "I've lost my motivation" monsters. *(Sound of victim screaming.)*

Oh boy, we know that mean old ogre, don't we?

We've lost ten pounds and we're strutting like John Stamos or Jane Fonda in *Barbarella*, until someone says, "Oh have you lost weight? I hadn't noticed."

Talk about a diet kill. It's enough to make you want to run home and eat a dozen Abazabas.

How many times have we done this...been destroyed by the "I've lost my motivation monster?"

We've given up too soon. Or we've taken all that weight off only to put it all back on—and then some?

Well, were done with that old way of doing things!

Time to get rid of the "I lost my motivation" monster!

You are now the new you, and your utility belt (which is now two notches tighter) is stuffed with new tools that will actually work. Should the dreaded "I lost my motivation" monster make its appearance, you will remember to K.I.S.S. and the 80/20 Plan.

Now, like Gandalf holding back the Bairog, take a broad stance facing down the refrigerator door, holding your wooden spoon as your staff, and shout, "You shall not pass!" (If others are asleep, just whisper it.)

As the "new you" you now know that *you will* take that weight off—and not just take it off but *keep it off!* Because right now, this very instant, you are already doing it! To stay on this glorious new path, here are a few tips:

HOW DO I STAY MOTIVATED?

Step 1 – Keep your expectations realistic

You've lost some weight. Your inner "hot babe" (or "stud muffin," if you're a guy) is emerging. Way righteously cool you!

However, you will overeat again.

You will likely binge again.

It's important you recognize that *you will slip up.*

If you assume you'll be in control for the rest of your life, when you do falter (and you will), you will label it as a "failure," and you will feel bad. And, as you learned in the beginning of this book, feeling bad triggers the urge to seek comfort—which we do by eating—and seeking comfort through food puts you right back in that eating cycle—which is a place you don't want to be.

So your *new* realistic expectations are: You will pig out. You will likely overdo it at the holidays. *And that's okay* because...

...staying healthy and thin is not a destination. It's a journey.

It is—as you've probably heard so many times before—a lifestyle, not a behavior. It is a complete makeover of not only what you eat and how much you move, but the very words you say to yourself. It is transformation from inside to outside, not the other way around.

With realistic expectations in place, when you falter, you are going to give yourself some positive self-talk: "I overdid it on Thanksgiving, and that's okay, 'cause

I'm back on track today with my new "K.I.S.S.-able plan," of parking the car far away from the mall and walking to the stores."

Or…

"I totally overdid it with the free samples at the grocery store. But that's okay, 'cause I'm gonna take the stairs instead of the elevator when I get home. (And if my house doesn't have an elevator, I'm gonna build one, and that should *really* burn some calories!)"

Step Two: *Avoid* the Food Bomb whenever possible

The "Food Bomb" is also known as bingeing, a/k/a mindless eating, a/k/a over-indulging.

Our goal is not to eliminate the Food Bomb. That's not realistic. (And we're setting Realistic Expectations now—go us!) It *is* to *learn how to handle* the Food Bomb, because although Food Bomb might not be welcome at your next event, she's probably going to show. And since you can't spend your life like Dr. Richard Kimble, constantly running from Food Bomb, you're going to have to deal with her at some point. (Technically Richard was avoiding the cops and looking for a one-armed man. However, we're willing to bet the stress of losing his wife, being falsely accused, and having to wrongly avoid law enforcement caused him to encounter a few Food Bombs along the way.)

Now that we know we can't eliminate Food Bomb from our life, we are going to need tools to disarm her. We can do this by:

Redefining success

Did you know that success is not a given in the universe? What we mean by that is that we don't need success to live complete lives as human beings. The earth would still spin. The sun would still rise. The rain would still fall. (Unless you live in California. Grab your hairbrush, make like it's a microphone, and sing with us now: "It never rains in California, but girl, don't they warn you, it pours. Oh, it pours.")

"Success" is a man-made construct; it is fluid and can come to mean anything we want it to mean.

Understanding that you determine what success is, and that it's not a given, but it's more powerful than the Justice League (and they're pretty powerful, except for that one beatnik-y kind of character who didn't do anything but snap his fingers a lot and didn't even have a costume. We don't think being 1950s hip is a superpower. We never got that).

Think of that. Success can mean anything you want it to mean. *You*, not your neighbors, not what "they" tell you, not what magazines say. *You* are the sole arbiter of what is success.

To some, success is a home in Malibu. To others, success is a tiny house with no mortgage. Success is a reality we create, and *we can change it any time we wish*. It is not a given, which means *you can redefine success and feel less bad/more successful more often.*

In the dark days (before we brought our own special form of sunshine into your life), you might have thought success was taking the weight off, never putting it back on, and always being in control. The problem with that definition of success is that it isn't realistic. When you aren't "successful" you feel like a failure. When you feel like a failure, you eat, steering you right back down Eating Cycle Boulevard.

So, by the powers invested in us, we now proclaim your new version of success eating to be:

1. (Gong!) Your Food Bomb occurs with less regularity. She doesn't visit as often.

2. (Gong!) Your Food Bomb causes less damage to your program and mental health then she formerly did.

3. (Gong!) You recover from the Food Bomb's visits so much faster.

Isn't that a lovelier version of Success? You didn't fail!

Let us give you an example from Scott's life

It was the end of a day from Hell. I was trolling the kitchen looking for anything I could eat.

You know the feeling: Open the pantry and stare inside for a while, looking for something that will take away the frustration but not cause too much damage in the process. Not finding anything, you repeat the process with the refrigerator. Then it's back to the pantry, back to the fridge. It's as if if you repeat this pattern enough times, a zero-calorie one-pound chocolate bar will magically appear.

As a protection against my Food Bomb exploding too often, I've cleaned my environment of what I refer to as "red light foods," leaving only "yellow light foods," those foods that are usually safe. For example, a red light food for me is peanut butter. I will not bring it into my house because I will devour an entire jar in one sitting. A yellow light food is cereal—the high fiber kind that tastes like cardboard. I can totally leave that in my cupboard—or use it to fix my roof if it expires. (The cereal's date, not the roof.)

And that's what my eyes lit upon at the end of this truly heinous day: a box of high-fiber cereal.

So here I am staring at this box of grains, and I am faced with a choice: Do I accept victory over my old habits (yay for me, I don't have any red light foods in the kitchen to taunt me), or do I devour this box of high-fiber cereal like it's the Holy Grail?

I opted for the latter.

Yes. I, Scott "Q" Marcus, ate the *entire* box of high fiber cereal. *(Burp, belch—* uh-oh, excuse me!)

I learned two valuable lessons from this experience, and I shall pass them on to you:

> Lesson #1: Never ever *ever* eat a whole box of high fiber cereal! Oh my God! It will turn your system into a brick and force you to make sounds I would rather not repeat here.

> Lesson #2: Even though what I did is not the most optimum example of making healthy choices, the box of high-fiber cereal was less damaging to my progress than ice cream would have been. And—and this is a big "and"— this type of events does not happen to me as often as such events once did.

What is the moral of Scott's saga?

Notice what you *have* done. Don't belabor what you didn't do.

Celebrate *(not with food!)* each victory. As Thomas Edison said, "You learned 4,672 ways you don't want to do it again." (We're not sure he actually said *those* words because when he was writing it down, it was dark and his penmanship sucked, but we're sure they are pretty close.)

Understand how the Food Bomb works:

The Food Bomb doesn't come into our lives via a Food Zombie (as much as we'd sometimes like to say it does).

Nope. We do not overeat because the Food Zombie comes into our living room on a dark stormy night and attacks us. We're not sitting on our couch, minding our own business, watching our favorite *Twilight Zone* reruns when *roarrrrrrrr,* the Evil Food Zombie schleps out of our TV. "Brains, must make them eat braaaainnnns (and other red light foods)" says Food Zombie.

"No!" says us. "Go away!"

We try to run. We call for help.

But the Food Zombie's will is just too strong for poor, weak us. And despite our protestations, we are *forced* to consume a pound of cheddar and a pint of Häagen Dazs (with whipped cream and rainbow sprinkles.)

No, that's not how it works.

Should we analyze it in slo-mo, what we would actually see is that:

Poor Baby Boomer us was slowly being squeezed with not one, not two, but a series of detonators. Detonators (you probably guessed) are like triggers that ignite our eating habit. However, whereas triggers are emotional, detonators are situational. Detonators go off at a certain time, or place, that makes us think of eating. For some people, a detonator might be watching late night TV; for others it could be a holiday dinner. (More times than not, detonators and triggers work together to create the perfect storm of overeating.)

The Food Bomb goes off when we have been hit by several detonators in a somewhat short period of time.

That's so important, we're going to recap that: The food bomb goes off only when several detonators are in place.

So let's look at what we mean by detonators:

(Mission Impossible *music would be great here)*

It's late into the evening. (Detonator One goes off.)

(Tick, tick, tick)

You are alone. Finally! (Detonator Two ignites.)

(Tick! tick! tick!) You're tired. (Detonator Three sizzles.)

(TICK, TICK, TICK)

You turn on the TV when you know you ought to go to bed. (Detonator Four explodes.) You're in your PJs. (Detonator Five explodes.)

(TICK! TICK! TICK!)

You haven't yet brushed your teeth. (Detonator Six) There's an availability of the right kind of food…and….

BOOM!

None of these events on its own is enough for the Food Bomb to explode. However, put them all together, and you're toast (with butter spray—after all, you are watching your weight).

Triggering the Food Bomb

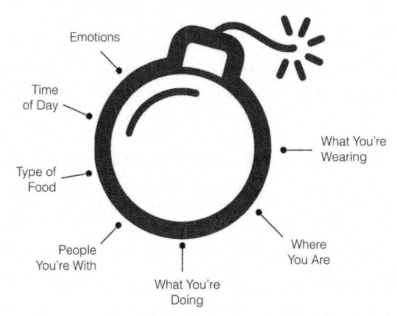

Emotions

Time of Day

Type of Food

People You're With

What You're Doing

Where You Are

What You're Wearing

It takes multiple Detonators to ignite the Food Bomb.

The good news is, you don't have to get rid of all the Detonators to disarm the Food Bomb. You must, however, get rid of enough Detonators to prevent the Food Bomb from exploding. You don't have to clean your house of all temptation by selling your television, throwing away all your comfy PJs, and brushing your teeth until the enamel is worn off. All you need do is remove one or two of those Detonators, and you'll be fine!

In those few moments when the detonators are sizzling, do something else. Put yourself into a new environment. It's so much easier to change your patterns *before* you have your head buried in the fridge.

Let's Play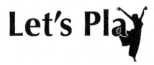

Ever watch *CSI?* Or maybe *Miami CSI?*

Well, now we're going to be in *Baby Boomer CSI*.

First thing you're gonna have to do is put on your pretend Hazmat suit. Then we want you to pull your pretend hood over your head. Now change your name to something action-y like Blaze Hill.

Okay, so it's the episode called "Late Night TV."

You're at home, and your phone rings. It's the Sergeant from the Bomb Squad. You're needed right away!

You're Detective Blaze. You knew this was coming. That's why you're already in your bomb gear.

You arrive on the scene to find a Food Bomb is about to go off! Oh no, this could be the end of life as we know it.

The Sarge says, "Hill, it's up to you. You've got to defuse this—"

You suck in a breath of courage and...

WRITE DOWN: a detailed description of what happened the last time you were confronted by a "Food Bomb."

WRITE DOWN: where you were, time of day, what you were doing, how long it had been since you last ate, and how you felt. Include every detail you can think of. The more details you remember, the more likely that the Food Bomb will not detonate next time.

With your list complete, read it over.

(Cue the ticker tape parade because you did save the city.)

Now write a plan. K.I.S.S. should that particular Food Bomb come your way again. A plan might be:

If your Food Bomb is late night eating when you're in your PJs: Floss teeth and brush as soon as dinner is over.

If your Food Bomb comes with you to parties: Bring healthy snacks and packs of gum to chew.

Now, put your plan where you can see it. If your Food Bomb is late night eating, put your plan by the couch to remind you. If your Food Bomb comes to parties, tape your plan to the front door so you can see it when you leave.

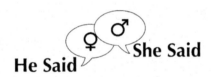

He Said / She Said

Today we take you back to days of yore..."Hi-ho, Silver, away!"
(*Cue:* William Tell Overture)

Sheriff Cindy saunters up the dusty street of a small Western Town in Anywhere, USA. Wooden sidewalks, two-story saloon—there's even tumbleweed rolling up the road.

Cindy wears her ten gallon hat, Dale Evans, fringed, cowgirl outfit, and a big lawman's badge.

Up runs Deputy Scott. Much to Scott's chagrin he looks more like Don Knotts than John Wayne.

Scott's heart races. His eyes are wide with fear. He's got bad news!

SCOTT:

Sheriff Cindy, Sheriff Cindy! We got trouble up in Peppermint Flats!

(Cindy nods, encouraging her deputy to go on.)

SCOTT:

(Scott spits) It's them Smucker's Brothers! They ain't happy. *(Scott spits)* They say that they're gonna food bomb Anywhere USA. And I think they mean business. *(Spits)*

CINDY:

Well, that ain't good, Scott, which means it's bad. Real bad. We're gonna have to pack up every last one of the town pantries, *and* Mister Chips Restaurant and Food Emporium, and move to Hershey Flats today!

SCOTT:

(spits) But is that realistic, Sheriff? Them Smucker's Boys will be here any minute—

CINDY:

(Sheriff Cindy considers this. Deputy Scott spits. The sheriff nods because she's got a plan.) You're right, Scott. It ain't realistic. We're gonna have to come up with a simpler plan. Tell me what you saw. Don't leave nothin' out.

SCOTT:

Well, Sheriff, I reckon I saw ten detonators! *(spit) (spit)*

CINDY:

(She smiles because she knows exactly what to do.) Well, Deputy, we beat back those varmints before. Means we can do it again. And they cain't bomb the town without them detonators—

SCOTT:

We got to steal all their detonators, Sheriff? *(spit)*

CINDY:

Nope. All we gotta do is defuse half.

SCOTT:

And they won't want to food bomb us no more?

CINDY:

Them Smucker's Brothers is bad hombres, and they're probably gonna wanna mosey on back one day. But we'll handle it then, too.

(Cindy smiles. One of her pearly whites actually twinkles. Our two heroes mount their horses and ride off into the sunset, knowing that because they created a realistic plan and defused not all but a few of the Smucker's Boys' detonators, their little town would once again be safe from harm.)

CHAPTER 9: HOW DO I STOP YO-YO DIETING?

The World According to Sc🌐tt

Ode to My Pants

Mirror, mirror in my room,
It's time to start my daily groom.
In previous days, we've oft locked horns,
Yet adorning myself will be different this morn

I've followed my diet so sure and sound,
My middle no longer as wide around.
Trying clothes from the closet, I used to hate.
With newfound pride, I don't hesitate

My favorite pants sit atop the list.
Praise for looks, once heard, has been sorely missed.
As I yank the trousers around my waist.
I foresee grand style, so I dress in haste.

But now my feelings become confused.
These pants? Too tight, leaving me bemused.
I inhale—deep breath—suck my stomach in.
I'm sure I've lost weight! Am I not yet thin?

I fuss, twist, and stretch, and I try to zip.
What's that sound I hear? Did the fabric rip?
Standing on my toes, am I somehow taller?
If I am, that should make my tummy smaller.

Lying on the bed. flat upon my back,
I accept I must try a diff'rent tack.
Then, with force, I fasten the snap in place
As exertion's sweat decorates my face.

Rolling carefully, I now try to rise.
But I can't help wond'ring about my size.
It seems the slacks are upon me now.
Breathing would be nice; but I'm not sure how

With stiff, shaky legs I stand up, unsure
If I have the strength left to reach the door.
Like a movie monster, I lurch, not walk,
With my pants so snug that I cannot talk.

"It's no use," I think, and remove my clothes.
I can breathe again! I can feel my toes!
As relief flows through me, my blood starts flowing.
These pants won't fit without loads of sewing.

It's a sad, sad truth, but I must admit
If I wear these pants then I cannot sit.
I'm exhausted, tired, and feeling blue.
Maybe I'm not yet a 32.

We were never very good with our trusty Duncan yo-yo. It would yo down but refused to yo back up again.

So it's kind of ironic that we're so damn proficient at yo-yo dieting, isn't it?

Yo-yo dieting happens because we have lost our motivation and returned to old habits to comfort us. It's as simple as that.

Old habits never die. They just go into a deep freeze, from which we can thaw them out whenever we need them.

When we are motivated, we are able to keep the freezer (probably avocado green or hunter's gold—ew!) at the right temperature. As our motivation wanes, old habits—which were designed to comfort us, remember?—start to warm up. Little by little, they warm our tired bones, and before we know it, we're back where we were.

Therefore, to prevent yo-yo dieting, we have to stay motivated.

Ah, but how do we *get* motivated when we're not?

To regain motivation, we need to set a meaningful—small—achievable—*small*—well-defined—**small**—goal that *we know* we can achieve. (Did we mention it has to be small?). Size matters here—and we're talking about size of the goal, not clothing size—because if our goal is too big it will overwhelm us, and bring up our triggers to eat. And we will give up.

Let's take an example:

We've set the goal: "We want to lose weight."

That's an awesome goal. Yay for us!

Except...

Uh oh. Our goal isn't clearly defined, is it? "I want to lose weight" could mean drop 5 pounds or it could mean drop 50. And are we talking about losing this ambiguous weight in a month? A week? A year?

You see? If our goal isn't well defined, specific, and measurable, how can we know when we get there? And if we don't know when we have arrived at "there," we begin to feel like a hamster in a wheel running and running and running and getting nowhere. We will then get frustrated and just give up. Exhausted and feeling like a failure, we are sucked back into the Eating Cycle, and voila—we are yo-yo dieting.

Let's Play

It's time to get out your journal and pen.

Write down ten healthy eating/staying fit goals. We want you to make them as specific as possible. Make them small, so that they can be accomplished in one day. Be sparklingly clear. And put in a deadline. Finally, write down how you will feel once you hit that goal.

So Cindy and Scott's goal might look like this:

We would like to write two pages of our book this Tuesday.

(Do you see how specific and small that is?)

We will feel joyous. And proud.

The golden ticket of motivation

Do you remember that movie, *Willy Wonka and the Chocolate Factory*? (Not the Johnny Depp one, but the real one, the "good" one, with Gene Wilder.) Anyway, in the movie, five kids each win a golden ticket and get to go to the chocolate factory. Well, "Oompa loompa, doopity do!" That golden ticket was something every kid, including those watching the movie, wanted to win. If you won, that ticket could make all your dreams come true. Wow!

And isn't that just how we look at becoming motivated to lose weight? We flit about, trying this and that, believing that Willy Wonka will drop down from the sky and hand us our "Golden Motivation Ticket." Ticket firmly in our hands, we will happily go on our diet.

We hate to burst your childhood bubble, but Topo Gigio wasn't a real mouse, gasoline isn't 25 cents a gallon anymore, Elvis is sadly no longer in the building, and real life isn't like the movies. (We know, right? That's so unfair.) Motivation doesn't happen that way.

Motivation is not an external force that's given to us like the prize in a Cracker Jacks Box. Rather, it is an internal force that is completely in our control. We bring on motivation—or send it away—whenever we choose to. We manifest our own motivation.

To *get* motivated, we must *create* motivation.

We know: That's backward from what you've been taught. (Us too.) But when we finally understood that motivation didn't come *before* action, it came *from* action, what a difference it made in maintaining our weight loss and ending yo-yo dieting.

Let's Play

Rip out one sheet of paper from your notebook.

Now rip that piece of paper into ten smaller pieces of paper. Go on, rip! Don't get all "grown-up-y" on us and get out your safety scissors (which never worked worth beans anyway) and cut the paper into ten even smaller pieces. (Unless you're OCD like us and cutting up paper makes you happy. Then go on. We give you full permission. Cut away.)

Lay out your pieces in front of you. Admire how pretty they are.

Get out your pen, and on each piece of paper write a word that you associate with being motivated. Here are a few we came up with:

- Empowered
- Enthused
- Excited
- Charged up (Okay, that's two words)
- Happy
- Powerful
- Confident
- Positive

Outasight! Hang onto those pieces of paper. Maybe put them in a drawer or envelope, but keep them nearby, because we're going to be using them again later in the chapter.

How does motivation feel?

It feels great, doesn't it? We feel empowered. Strong. In control. Feeling motivated feels like nothing can stop us now. It's so energizing, we feel like Mary Tyler Moore throwing her hat in the air and singing, "You're gonna make it after all."

But sometimes it doesn't feel that way. Sometimes it doesn't feel like the Beatles landing in New York to standing ovations. Often it's hiding in the shadows, whispering quietly. And if you want to hear it, you have to *really* listen. But you have the power to turn up the volume. Either screaming or whispering, motivation is in your control.

Here's the thing: Significant change doesn't begin due to motivation. That's upside-down. In fact, all significant change comes because of a combination of fear, force, and/or pain.

That's so important, we'll repeat it: **All significant change is generated by fear, force, and/or pain.**

No one wakes up one morning, takes inventory of her/his life, and says, "Wow! Everything is working out just like I wanted. Let me see how I can change it." Rather they arise to a lifestyle suffocating them in a bucketload of hurt. Because they are desperate (some call it "hitting rock bottom"), they are willing to try something— *anything*—different. That psychic—even physical—pain is the seed of change. So the actual feelings that ignite self-improvement are:

- Fear
- Frustration
- Sadness
- Shame
- Guilt
- Anxiety
- Worry
- Resignation

That list sure doesn't look like motivation, does it? However, out of the need to escape those feelings, we are propelled to take action. Due to the pain and the resulting different action we take, we feel different. *That* is motivation revving up.

It is important to realize that: fear, force, or pain are actually what inspire us to change; it's not joy, happiness and strength.

Phew! Take that in a moment. Let that resonate. We have been yo-yo dieting because we have gotten discouraged about reaching our goal. We have fallen back on unhealthy eating patterns and stayed there because motivation didn't come as we thought it would with feelings of "You can do this!" "You're a winner!" and "Whip Inflation Now!"

You see? Yo-yo dieting wasn't totally your fault. You've been misinformed all these years.

But now you are the new you (even if you insist on wearing Earth Shoes.) And you are ready to stop yo-yo dieting. You are ready to take that weight bull by the horns, wrestle it to the ground, and say "No more!"

Motivation gets a whole new look

So now that we've taken the golden shine off motivation, let's look at how *real* motivation looks:

We can't get down on the floor to play with our grandchildren because we won't be able to get back up again. Ouch! We take action: we sign up for a water aerobics class to get in shape.

Our spouse no longer finds us attractive because we've stopped taking care of ourselves. Big ouch! We take action: we start doing our walking again.

The doctor says we have diabetes, and if we don't take off at least 20 pounds we'll be put on shots and meds. Mondo mega-sized ouch! We take action: we buy this book.

(Which, in all honesty, was a brilliant decision for someone in so much pain. We are really impressed with you. We were just talking about you a few minutes ago. Scott turned to Cindy and said, "Isn't he/she impressive?"

Cindy said, "Yes, he/she is, but, I don't think he/she will really believe we had this conversation since we don't even know which gender he/she is."

Scott thought about that for a moment and then, in his best Emily Litella voice, replied, "Never mind.")

It was fear, force, or pain that marched into our lives wearing cleats and shooting an Uzi. Fear, force, or pain made us act. So we start: tracking our food *or* weighing and measuring portions *or* going to a support group *or* taking a daily walk.

Yes, it is one small step, but it's a "giant step for..." you. (That's an Apollo reference. We sat here and argued about using an Apollo reference because you might not get it, and Cindy didn't really love Buzz Aldrin, which confused Buzz and hurt his feelings, but we figured you guys are smart and we didn't need to point out it was an Apollo reference.) And because we have taken this one small but *different* action, we get at least one *different* result, which feels so much better. We sigh and glow in our success for a moment. (It's important that you take that moment to sigh and glow, to acknowledge that success. Don't gloss over it; don't get all grownuppy and dismiss it. Celebrate it!)

Now motivation wants to come back. You've made it safe and welcome. We take another small and different action in the right direction. We feel even better. Maybe we drop a pound (not 50), or the ache in our back diminishes (even if we can't work the parallel bars yet), or we can put on a pair of pants without having to lie on the bed to fasten the snap.

When we focus on these new fledgling results, fresh feelings arise:

- Enthusiasm
- Excitement
- Charged up-ness
- Happiness
- Powerfulness
- Confidence

Dare we say it? We are motivated! We feel happier and empowered by *our* choices, not by something from outside us. We created this motivation by the actions *we* did. Now motivated, like Forrest Gump running across the country, we don't stop. We have the desire to seek out stronger and more effective behaviors to continue getting those empowering results. And we're back to that positive self talk we discussed way back at the beginning of this book.

The bottom line is that motivation does not lead behavior. It follows it.

So, right now, let's make a pledge. Stand up and put your right hand in the air. Put your left hand over your heart.

(Hmmm, wait, you won't be able to read the pledge if we do that. Okay, so just stand up. Don't tell us you were already standing up—no one reads standing up.)

Come on....

Others are waiting, you know. We can't continue with this book until you do it.

There, doesn't that feel better?)

(ahem) Back to Our Pledge—

Repeat after me. "I—insert your name–

(Don't be cute and say out loud "Insert Your Name." We we've heard that before. It's gotten old.)

...promise to stop looking for that Golden Ticket of Motivation and recognize that it's a fallacy and never really existed. I promise that when I feel fear, force, or pain, I will acknowledge them as catalysts to take actions (which will not include eating). I will then take a moment to feel proud of myself and enjoy feeling motivated."

You can now sit back down.

Remember, initially, what inspires us to take action looks like that moody, irritable friend that you want to run from but can't. She nudges and nips and bothers us until we take action. Action taken, we start to feel better. The better we feel, the more action we want to take. The more action we take, the better we feel. Motivation now looks prettier and prettier. She's happy and encouraging, and we like having her around. After all, we created her.

Let's Play

We're gonna make a "Motivation Jar."

You will need: a mason jar, or a shoe box, or a container of some kind, another ten pieces of paper, and a pen. Stickers, glitter glue, and paint are optional.

1. Get out those pieces of paper with the empowering words you wrote.

2. Read the first one. Now take out one of your blank pieces of paper and write down an action helping you toward your weight loss goals that goes with that feeling of empowerment. In other words, write down what you would need to do to make you feel that way.

Let's say we wrote down the word "happy." Our action of empowerment might be to look up some new light recipes and make one.

Let's say we wrote down the word "strong." Our action of empowerment might be do five sit-ups every night for a week.

Let's say we wrote down the word "confident." Our action of empowerment might be sit up straight at the dinner table.

Do you see what we mean? Motivation is an action inspired by a feeling.

3. Write down an empowering action for each feeling.

4. Now on your jar write the words "Motivation Jar." If you want, decorate your container. You can put stickers on it or paint it purple. Make the box as inspiring as you like.

5. Put your empowerment actions inside the jar.

6. Take out one of the empowerment actions from the jar whenever you feel that "I'm not motivated monster" return. Read it.

7. Do the action.

8. Think of a new feeling and a new action to go with it. Write that down, put it in the jar.

9. Leave the jar visible. (Maybe even put a Motivation Jar in each room.)

10. Pat yourself on the back. Job well done.

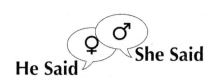

He Said 　She Said

(Now, when we think "motivation," we think of that amazing scene from *Rocky* where he's running up the steps in Philadelphia and tossing his fists into the air—oh come on, you know the one. Admit it. Every time you walk up a flight of steps you sing the *Rocky* theme song.)

So in honor of *Rocky* and all things motivational, we give you— *SCOTTY*

(*Scotty is standing at his counter. He's got a couple of raw eggs, unbroken, in one hand, a glass in the other. In comes Cindy. She looks a lot like Burgess Meredith, beanie on her head, straggly beard. She's worn but determined to make Scotty the champ she knows he is. Scotty cracks the eggs into the glass. He brings the raw ick up to his mouth to drink—*)

CINDY:

Scotty! Whatcha think youse doin'?

SCOTTY:

(*who sounds so much like Sylvester Stallone it's kind of freaky*) Yo. Cindy. Go away. You ain't wanted here.

CINDY:

I ain't leavin' you, Scotty. You heard what dat doctor said. You gonna be lean and mean. If you wanna crap thunder you gotta eat better.

SCOTTY:

No. I'se got to train!

CINDY:

No, dem raw eggs is a heart attack waitin' to happen. At your age, you got to watch dat cholesterol. Eat an egg white omelet, a few avocados, 'cause dose are da healthy oils.

(*Scotty looks at his egg goop. He looks at Cindy. The* Rocky *theme slowly, quietly rises*)

SCOTTY:

Youse right, Cindy.

(*Like the champ he is, Scotty washes the raw eggs down the sink. He opens the fridge and starts making a healthy egg white omelet as the* Rocky *theme kicks into high gear.*)

CHAPTER 10: BRINGING BACK MOTIVATION

The World According to Sc⊕tt

When on vacation, I dress quicker than my wife, having less hair and therefore less of a need to blow-dry it. With the extra time, I find myself waiting for her at the hotel restaurant.

"What will it be this morning?" asks the waitress.

Studying the menu, I am engaged in a fierce internal debate between "responsible" (fresh fruit) and "desirable" (hash browns, bacon, omelet, croissant). Adult overrules inner child, and I order "something light," oatmeal.

Momentarily a bathtub-size basin arrives. Submerged in thick, rich cream, smothered with a brown, syrupy liquid of melted maple sugar, is my hot cereal. Realizing it's too late to ask for non-fat milk and sugar on the side, I reassure myself the faux pas won't harm my diet. Everyone knows unintended calories don't count; fat cells realize the error and disregard the weight gain.

The waitress places a platter of sugary condiments on the table before leaving. At first, I am inclined to resist them, but re-evaluate. Maybe this is a local tradition; it would be rude to offend our hosts. Besides, I'm on vacation; it's almost an edict that one sample new foods while traveling.

Rationale safely locked in place, to others I must appear to be an alchemist developing a brew in a cauldron. I put in butter, honey, cream, yogurt (three flavors), strawberry jam, grape jelly, raw sugar, and cashews. I would mix in yet more, but I'm concerned the table will buckle under the weight of my "light snack." The embarrassment could put a damper on my day.

Sipping down the concoction, I refill the bowl with sugary additives each time it drops below the rim. After a few iterations, I'm unsure any original oatmeal remains, but I continue to add more flavorings as the rainbow swirl of reds, yellows, purples, and browns has me on a full-tilt sugar buzz, and rational thinking is no longer an option.

My wife arrives, sliding into the booth as I clean the remains of the bowl. The inclination to use my finger like a spatula and scrape the edges is overruled in favor of a more mature demeanor.

She looks at the plate, "You ate already? I thought we were going to have breakfast together?"

"It was nothing—just a small bowl of oatmeal to hold me over."

HOW DO WE REDISCOVER MOTIVATION?

When we've lost our way, and the dreaded "I lost my motivation" monster comes a-barkin' on our doorstep like an unwanted mongrel mutt, don't worry, motivation didn't move out! Motivation is just upstairs in the attic listening to all your old 45s (probably putting a penny on the tone arm so they don't skip).

But the appearance of that unwanted mutt is a sign:

You have stopped doing the behaviors that brought on Motivation in the first place. And it is time for (drum roll, please)…

"I Do"

Since we are with our body our entire life (except of course for some of those out-of-body experiences we might have had in college), it stands to reason that we need to treat it like our significant other. To that end, we would now like to present to you, your wedding—to your body.

(We know, we know—this is a little strange. But just go with it.)

Do you, sweet Boomer, take this body of yours for richer or poorer, in sickness and in health, through Ben and Jerry's binges and grapefruit diets? Do you solemnly swear to stand by your body when it wears leg warmers and mini-skirts and pink hair? Will you honor and keep it when it refuses to get up and go to yoga, or when it limbos at your niece's wedding when it should have waltzed? Then say "I do."

"I do. We do. We, me and my body, are married."

Congrats. You have just committed to the most significant relationship of your life!

(Scott and Cindy throw rice!)

Now what?

Well as many of us know, getting married and staying married are two very different things. Staying married means we're gonna face a lot of crap together. And like any other relationship, ours—the one we each have with our body—isn't always gonna go as we want it to. But you're still in love and don't want to quit each other.

With any long-term relationship, you will periodically have "issues." If you have a problem with your significant other, do you simply say, "Jane, you ignorant slut," and close off the conversation? No, that's not going to help. Do you give up and get a divorce at the first sign of problems? Probably not, even though you might consider it. No, if you want it to work, you expect that there will be bumps along the way, and you also expect that you will work them out. It might not be comfortable or fun, but you're committed to making it work.

That commitment will get you to your goal weight and help you keep a healthy lifestyle until death do you part. So if you are at loggerheads with your body, you will need tools to get the two of you back on track.

We want you want you to slow down and "Think 1st."

Note that we didn't spell it "think first."

"Think 1st" is an acronym: a healthy mnemonic device to help you remember something; you know like when we learned the colors of the rainbow in school: ROY G BIV or how to remember musical notes on a page: Every Good Boy Deserves Favor.

Think 1st is:

Pick **1** task.

Make it **S**imple.

Focus on **T**oday.

Think 1st ties everything together in one neat little package. And guess what: It also reminds us to think before we act.

When we get stuck, it's because we've gone too big. We've forgotten that whatever we do has to be simple *and* easy. Remember that?

Since we know that losing weight is already a simple thing to do—eat less, move more – it stands to reason that our plan of attack has gotten complicated. It's no longer simple. We've probably blown it up into this big old gigantic mass of gears and cogs and messy stuff and we've become so overwhelmed we don't know where to begin.

(Poor beleaguered, crazed us)

We must then "come back, Shane" to the land of Easy. To get to this wonderful valley where things make sense and you can get back on your program, you will need to Think 1st:

- Pick **1** task
- Make it **S**imple
- Focus on **T**oday

Pick 1 task

Pick one—not a bunch, just one single solitary behavior that you know you can do because you've done it before. Usually, the first action that comes to mind is the best one.

How do you know if the task you've chosen is too small? That's a great question, Grasshopper. If the result from doing that action will leave you exactly where you were before you did the action, it's too small because—let's be honest—nothing changed. You didn't do anything. Aside from that, there is no "too small."

Make it Simple

Ask yourself, could I do this right now without having to go anywhere else, purchase anything, or call anyone? If not, go back to "Pick one task" and go even smaller. There's actually a principle of simplicity summed up by something called "Occam's razor" which states, "All things being equal, the simplest solution tends to be the best one." (We don't know who Occam is or what it has to do with shaving, but the advice cannot be denied.)

Focus on Today

You have chosen your task. You made sure it's in your control and, just like the Nike commercial, do it! Don't put it off. Don't pass GO and wait for that $200 (which won't buy you much anyway). Instead, make a promise to yourself that you will do it before your head hits the pillow tonight.

If you're not willing to do it, it's a sure sign what you have chosen is too big, too complicated, or is not your goal. Take the task and continue to make it smaller and/or simpler until you know you'll do it.

The coolest part about our handy, dandy Think 1st System is that you're not making any long-term commitment to your Think 1st plan of the moment.

If you try a Think 1st plan and it doesn't work? No worries.

1.   By Thinking 1st you have gotten unstuck from whatever gluey substance was holding you back.

2.   You can try a new Think 1st plan later or tomorrow. Yay for you!

Let's Play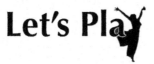

"It's Howdy Doody time. It's Howdy Doody time..."

(Not really. But we love the following game so much fun we just felt like we had to sing something.)

For this game you will need your journal and a pen. However, if you want to really go all out, get yourself a plain index card (without any lines). Whatever color floats your boat on the card works for us. You are going to make...

The "I Promise" card

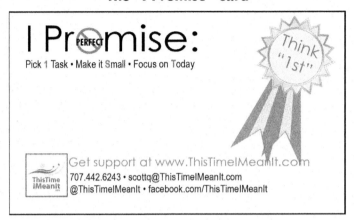

(Or if you if you'd like one made by us, which is printed all professional, you can print out a sheet of our pre-made I PROMISE CARDs, which you can cut out. All you have to do is go to www.ThisTimeIMeanIt.com/downloads and download it.)

If you have craft in your fingers and a song in your heart and want to make your own card, here's how you do it:

1.   Write "I Promise…" in dark, large letters, along the top, just like you see in the example.

2.   Now, without thinking, answer the following question and write it on the card.

"The very next thing I need to do to feel happier, healthier, or more successful is _____"

(If it takes you more than about 30 seconds, you're thinking too hard. Make it easy and simple. Just write it on the card.)

3.   Put the card on your refrigerator or pantry or computer monitor or mirror— somewhere where you can see it.

4.   As you place your I Promise card in its *very visible* place of honor, take a moment and make a commitment to yourself that you will make sure to read and think about your promise for one minute.

What's totally bitchin' about the I Promise card is you can make it business card size – which is 2 by 3.5 inches. You can put it in your wallet and look at it wherever you go.

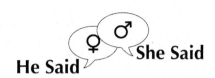

He Said / She Said

Here's the story of a man named Scott, who was busy with diets of his own.

He was one man....

You guessed it, in this very special episode of He Said/She Said, Scott Brady and his daughter, Cindy Brady, must learn to Think 1st *(laugh track)*.

(We hear that dorky '70s music as Cindy Brady comes running into the Brady living room. Mr. Scott Brady is sitting on the sofa, reading the paper.)

CINDY BRADY:

Daddy! Daddy!

SCOTT BRADY:

Yes. Cindy. What is it?

(Laugh track for no apparent reason)

CINDY BRADY:

Alithe thez I have to eat my lunch. Mommy thez I have to do my homework. But I want to pound Bobby in the fathe. What do I do?

SCOTT BRADY:

Now, Cindy.... Nobody likes a lot of information, because too much information means your information is not really informed. And an uninformed idea only informs the world that you're not really informing us of any useful information.

CINDY BRADY:

Huh?

(Laugh track again. We still don't know why.)

SCOTT BRADY:

Remember we always Think First.

CINDY BRADY:

You're right, Daddy.

(Cindy skips offstage to pound Bobby.)

BOBBY:

(O.S.) Ow! Geez! Cindy, quit....

The Brady Bunch, The Brady Bunch. That's how Scott and Cindy became the Brady Bunch.... And how you remember to always Think 1st!

CHAPTER 11:
BYE BYE MISS AMERICAN (LOW CAL) PIE

The World According to Sc⊕tt

A few months ago, I lamented the fact that I would soon be turning sixty. Well, try as I might to deny the inevitable, September 28 has arrived. I am now officially entering my seventh decade.

Also, as I mentioned, I grok that there are people looking at sixty in their rear view mirrors, most likely shaking their heads, thinking, "Come on, Scott. Get over it!" Yet I remind these naysayers that this is the oldest I've ever been. My wife, in an attempt to be supportive, I presume, has been espousing, "Remember, today is the youngest you'll be for the remainder of your life."

Hmmm... I don't know whether that's comforting or not. But what can I say? She's a child in her fifties. She'll learn.

So I went to the doctor for a check-up. They checked my weight ("You've lost a few pounds since last year." Yay!) and blood pressure ("We need to watch that." Sigh.)

Then came my height.

I'm going to be vulnerable here, so be gentle with your judgment, okay? Most of my adult life, I've lied about my height, insisting I'm a towering 5′ 9″ when I'm actually a diminutive 5′ 8″. One might rightly wonder why that extra inch matters so much to my obviously frail psyche, and that's a fair question. Yet, the honest reply is: I haven't a clue. Maybe it's a guy thing—who knows? Anyway, of late, with newfound maturity, I've finally come to grips with the reality that major league basketball is not going to come calling and have accepted my actual stature.

So, it's one of nature's practical jokes that I find out I've shriveled to five-seven and a half!

"What's that about?" I asked the doctor.

"It's normal."

"Really? Can't I do something about it? Stretch more? Hang upside-down?"

"No, it's age appropriate."

That's a weird phrase. I've always considered "age appropriate" to define behaviors rather than physical traits.

"So, anything else I should know about?" he asked, pulling up a chair.

I pulled out my written list (really) of the aches, pains, and concerns I'm experiencing. After all, I'm given only fifteen minutes; I'm going to get my money's worth. First on my inventory is a nagging ache in my wrist. He inspected both arms, gently poking and prodding, and informed me, "It's tendonitis, nothing serious."

"What causes that?"

"Probably just your age. If it doesn't get better, come back and we'll see what we can do."

Next anxiety: My skin isn't so smooth anymore. There are bumps and blemishes popping up almost as rapidly as the hairs on my head that aren't vanishing are turning gray. I pointed out the more dastardly offenders.

Yet again, my fears vaporized. "Nothing out of the usual. It's not cancer, and I see no cause for concern." Of course *he* doesn't see any cause for trepidation. It's not *his* arms that have the texture of sun-dried tomatoes.

"Is there anything I can do about it?" I asked. Surely, a doctor in the golden age of medical miracles has some sort of potion one can smear on and restore vitality and youth. After all, this is the future we foresaw in the sixties. I mean, we don't have flying cars and food pills, but there oughta be something we can do about turkey-skin-arms.

"Not really. It's age appropriate."

Yikes! Again with that cursed expression. I didn't use it that much when I was raising my kids.

So I left his office; satisfied that I'm in "age appropriate" good health but still fuming about the changes I'm experiencing—a definite reminder that aging is mandatory but maturity is optional.

Senior moments

Have you ever walked from one room to the other to do something—maybe put away a book, or get your keys, or turn off a light—you know, something really mundane—and in the five seconds it takes you to get to the other room, you've totally blanked on what it was you were going to do? You find yourself standing in the center of the room, scratching your head and muttering, "Now why was I coming in here?"

That was not our problem in writing this book. Actually, it's been the opposite. What began as a detailed outline of all the things we wanted to share with you has morphed into this huge list.

We wanted to share *everything* with you.

(Like that time when Cindy was seven and threw Scott's shoes outside, and he had to chase after them, which made him awfully mad but was really Cindy's way of helping him with his weight loss. Or when Scott learned that Cindy used to slap herself and get red skin and then tell their parents Scott was hurting her so he'd get in trouble. And when Scott was then able to prove he wasn't doing it and their parents stopped believing Cindy, so he really did slap her. Jeeze, we were cruel little kids, weren't we?)

Okay, wait, what were we saying? Oh, right.

But then we realized, if we shared *everything,* this book would rival *War and Peace* in length. Since it became impractical to cram our little tome with every fix and foible we've learned over the years, and because—dear Boomer—we know you know all there is to know about eating programs and such, and you are way too busy for us to bombard you with pages and pages of information, we've included only the easiest and the simplest things to implement.

Still, what final pearls of wisdom can we share with you? Or what is the yummiest icing on the cake…or the (low-fat) crème de la crème?"

The ten-minute rule

When you're overwhelmed or you feel defeated and you've lost your mojo, and you're about to cross over into the land of no return (a loaded cupboard), just wait ten minutes before you decide what to do next.

That's it.

It may seem like such a simple (there's that word again) thing to do, but the results will be amazing.

HOW DOES THE TEN-MINUTE RULE WORK?

- It's specific. Ten little minutes. You can tell if you've achieved your objective before the next commercial break.
- It's easy.
- It's simple. You don't need any plans or tools. It can be done from anywhere at any time.
- It's empowering. It puts the control within you. You take the action.
- It's realistic. You know you can do it if you want.

Two tips for the ten-minute rule

1. Don't set a timer. Should you be distracted and the timer bell dings, you'll respond like Pavlov's pooch and think about eating again. Not what you're going for.

2. Do not "white-knuckle" the ten minutes. The ten-minute rule is designed to get you away from emotional anxiety. (Isn't that why you're doing the ten minute rule in the first place? So you won't fall victim to the Food Cycle?) Walk away instead. It's so much better for you on so many levels.

Remember, feelings move through us quickly; chances are, in less than a minute or seven, whatever you're feeling will change. So all we really need to do is slow down our habit long enough to allow reason in; we will then—more times than not—make a great decision. Just try it for ten minutes and see how it works.

Let's Play

For our final game, you will need your journal and pen.
We want you to write down all the things you can accomplish in ten minutes.
You'd be surprised at how powerful that little block of time is.
Here are a few ideas:

1. Dance
2. Make a salad
3. Write an email
4. Walk around a very short block
5. Climb up and down a few flights of stairs
6. Hug your honey.
7. Ask your child about their day.
8. Return a phone call.
9. Toss a frisbee with your dog.
10. Write ten things that are awesome about you.

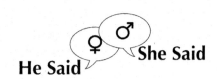

He Said She Said

"We're so glad we had this time together, just to share a laugh and sing a song. .Seems we just get started and before you know it, it's the time we have to say so long."

No games. No silly scripts. This one is just gonna be Scott and Cindy.

CINDY:

Wow. This has been amazing for me.

SCOTT:

Me too.

CINDY:

Thank you so much for letting me share in this journey.

SCOTT:

Thanks for all your help.

CINDY:

My pleasure.

SCOTT:

And thanks, dear Boomer, for your strength…

CINDY:

And courage…

SCOTT:

And willingness to change.

CINDY:

We're really excited for you! And we know you're gonna do this.

SCOTT:

You already are!

The World According to Sc🌐tt

(ONE MORE TIME)

As children, we couldn't wait to get older. We couldn't wait to hit that magical, double digit age of ten. And then every year from then on, it just seemed like something new and exciting was around the bend.

At thirteen, it was my Bar Mitzvah. Sixteen brought a driver's license; eighteen ushered in the newly earned right to vote; twenty-one got celebrated with (too much) champagne. There was always another reason to move on to the next year. Bring 'em on. Line 'em up! Don't stop!

However, as John Mellencamp lamented in, "The Real Life," "It's a lonely proposition when you realize/That there's less days in front of the horse/Than riding in the back of this cart." Aside from the fact that it should be "fewer days" (sorry, I couldn't resist), his lyrics are spot on. It's macabrely humorous that as soon as one begins to realize he's on the downward slope of the hill, pumping the brakes in vain to avoid that inevitable *crash,* the thought of aging loses its wonder. Suddenly, we don't want to grow older. We want to slow time down. But it just seems to accelerate faster and before you know it, we're getting AARP brochures and worse yet, solicitations from the Neptune Society!

So yeah, sure, there's that "death thing" looming out there, which does cast a pallid gloom. Yet, spending my remaining years bemoaning a natural and unavoidable conclusion seems a pretty rotten way to live those very years.

I want to spend my time wrapping my brain around the cool things about getting older, so whenever yanked to the getting-older-sucks magnet, I can repel easier.

First, the hastening of time allows me to appreciate those "smaller moments," like sitting on a couch beside my wife (who is still a total babe to me even after twenty years together) reading; listening to the gleeful chortles of a toddler chasing a puppy; indulging in a red-yellow-gold sunset as it melts behind the ocean. They are such small things, and I never enjoyed them when I was building my career and growing my family.

Also, I don't care as much what others may think. I mean, I might not wear a Hawaiian shirt, checkered knee socks, and black wingtip shoes like my dad did, but with this age comes a way cool "This is me. Take it or leave it" attitude that I really like.

Never was I harsh, but now, with age, comes the wisdom about when to open my yap and when not to. Should I disagree with someone, my credo has evolved from "me first" to "compassion first." And I chose relationships that have real meaning for me now. I don't waste time with people who don't inspire or touch my heart, so the quality of my relationships—as with good wine or fine cheese—is richer because I am older and (hopefully) wiser.

AND CINDY SAYS

I'm not gonna wax philosophical like my big bro. (Though I totally agree with everything he just said.)

What I did want to say is that "I believe in you." And I know you can do this. It doesn't matter where you've been or what you've done in the past. That was then. And this is now. And this is your time because if you don't make these changes now, then when?

Our mom, Ruth, was obese her entire life. She battled weight like a warrior. Up and down she would go. And for most of her life she hated the body she lived in. She wouldn't go swimming, even though she loved the water, because she didn't want people to see her in a bathing suit. She always, always wore that layered look because it gave her a "longer look," and she wanted to hide her shape. (Even if it was 110 in the shade).

But here's the thing. Ruth was also brilliant. And beautiful. And one of the most talented women I have ever met. She was a rock. And she could make you see the world in a whole new way.

But none of that mattered to her. She was large, and for most of her life, she felt ashamed of who she was.

(Ah, but this story has a happy ending. Remember, I'm the bubbly one.)

When she turned sixty-five, Ruth realized that if she didn't lose her weight *now*, then when would she ever take it off?

So she returned to Nate Notchers with a commitment she'd never had before. That ticking clock that was growing louder by the day motivated her to change. Her age was the reason she returned to weight loss with a vengeance.

That's what's so awesome. It was her age that turned things around for her.

And boy, did she embrace the changes she needed to make, like the time she learned she had to "increase her activity." And she wanted music to help her on her way. Our sixty-something-year-old mom bought herself a Walkman (remember those?) and made mix-tapes and rocked out!

Her new size brought with it a confidence she'd never had. She met a hot sixty-something guy named Joe, and she giggled. And blushed.

Age didn't limit her, it expanded her. (But not her dress size. That shrank.)

And that's what I want for you. (For us.)

Let this age—whatever age you be—open up new possibilities. Realize that with age comes wisdom you didn't have fifteen or five or even one year ago. You can do this now. And now. And now. And....

From both of us, "May you age in a constant state of awe and wonder." (And remember, awe and wonder won't add to your weight by even one ounce! Go for it!)

The Baby Boomer's Groovy Playlist
(or appendix for you literary types)

1.   Hot Stuff, sung by Donna Summer, written by: Pete Bellotte, Harold Faltermeyer, Keith Forsey
2.   The Boys are Back in Town, sung by Thin Lizzy, written by Phil Lynett
3.   Y.M.C.A., sung by the Village People (young man) and written by Jacques Morali and Victor Willis
4.   Another Saturday Night, sung by Cat Stevens (this is the Sam Cooke song we mentioned, but we bet you knew it, huh?) and written by Sam Cooke. (Okay. All right. If you insist, you can have a point if you said the song was made famous by Sam. Yeesh!)
5.   I Just Want to Celebrate, sung by Rare Earth, written by Dino Fekaris and Nick Zesses
6.   Hot Legs, sung by Rod Stewart, written by Stewart and Gary Grainger
7.   Bicycle Race, sung by Queen (the champions my friend) and written by Freddie Mercury.
8.   Happy Days (theme song), sung by Jim Haas and written by Norman Gimble and Charles Fox.
9.   Let's Get Down Tonight, sung by KC and the Sunshine Band, written by Harry Wayne Casey and Richard Finch.
10.   Boogie "oogie oogie", sung by Taste of Honey and written by (yes, this song was actually written by someone), Fonce and Larry Mizell.
11.   McCarthur Park, sung by Donna Summer (yes, we get it, it was also made famous by Richard Harris, but this is the 70's version), written by Jimmy Webb.
12.   Ain't That a Shame, sung by Fats Domino, written by Fats and Dave Bartholomew
13.   You Can't Always Get What You Want, sung by the Rolling Stones, written by Mick Jagger and Keith Richards
14.   You Took the Words Right Out of My Mouth, sung by Meat Loaf (Cindy's husband's favorite) and written by Jim Steinman.
15.   Downtown, sung by Petula Clark and written by Tony Hatch
16.   Dance the Night Away, sung by Van Halen, written by: Alex, Michael and Eddie Van Halen, and David Lee Roth.
17.   Big Yellow Taxi, sung by Joni Mitchell and written by Joni.

18.   Money, sung by Pink Floyd, written by Roger Waters.
19.   Deuce, sung by Kiss, written (on a bus) by Gene Simmons
20.   Take the Long Way Home, sung by Super Tramp and writer by Rick Davies and Roger Hodgson.
21.   Show Me the Way, sung by Peter Frampton, written by Frampton.
22.   Follow Me, follow You, sung by Genesis, written by: Tony Banks, Phil Collins (huh) and Mike Rutherford
23.   Lady, sung by Lionel Ritchie and written by Kenny Rogers.
24.   You Make My Dreams Come True, sung by Hall and Oates, written by Hall, Oats and Sara Allen.
25.   I'm a Believer, sung by the Monkees, written by Neil Diamond.
26.   You Should be Dancing, sung by the Bee Gees, and written by: Barry, Robin and Maurice Gibb.
27.   Question, sung by The Moody Blues, written by Justin Hayward.
28.   (Sitting On) The Dock of the Bay, sung by Otis Redding, written by Redding and Steve Cropper.
29.   Workin' For a Living, sung by Huey Lewis and the News, written by: Scott Gibson, Christopher Hayes, Thomas Hopper, Victor Colla, Anthony Gregg and Carlo Cipollina
30.   Eve of Destruction, sung by Barry McGuire, written by P.F. Sloan.
31.   Oh Happy Day, sung by the Edwin Hawkins Singers, written by Hawkins (based on an 18th Century Hymn)
32.   One, sung by 3 Dog Night, written by Harry Nilsson
33.   It Never Rains in California, sung by Albert Hammond, written by Hammond.
34.   The Howdy Doody Theme Song, sung by the Peanut Gallery, written by Edward Kean (based the tune Ta Ra Ra Boom De Ay).
35.   The Brady Bunch Theme Song, sung by The Brady Bunch, written by Sherwood Schwartz
36.   American Pie, sung by Don McLean, written by McLean.
37.   Carol's Theme, sung by Carol Burnett and written by her husband, Joe Hamilton. (The snagging of her earlobe was a howdy to her grandma and she continued that tradition after her grandmother passed away.)
38.   Bat Out of Hell, sung by Meat Loaf, written by Jim Steinman (who considered it the ultimate car crash song).

About the Authors

Scott has lost 2,327 pounds – IF you add up all the weight he has lost (and regained) from childhood until he was 39, when he finally discovered the "secret to weight loss success" and dropped 70 pounds — which he has now maintained since the mid nineties. Therefore, he is jokingly referred to as a "THINspirational speaker" and his lively, upbeat presentations have been described as a "cross between nutrition 101, group therapy, and a southern revival." In addition to being an award-winning speaker, he is past president of the northern California chapter of the National Speakers Association, a syndicated newspaper columnist, as well as an author of eight

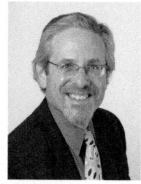

other books, and the founder of ThisTimeIMeanIt.com, a site to help fellow "recovering perfectionists" get past what holds them back. He lives with his wife in the Redwoods along the beautiful northcoast of California, and has been known to do presentations in exchange for good quality chocolate. (But he'll deny it.)

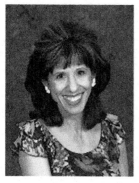

Cindy is used to working with a partner. She's co-written for Star Trek Deep Space Nine, spent five years on staff at Disney where she penned the biggest selling video in history, The Lion King II - Simba's Pride as well as many other animated features. She has over three dozen plays and musicals that are performed all across the globe. She's also the author of the non-fiction books Playdate, and The Ultimate Young Actor's Guide. She lives in Los Angeles with her husband, son, and quite possibly the greatest dog in the world.

CPSIA information can be obtained at www.ICGtesting.com
Printed in the USA
BVOW07s0601260216

437893BV00007B/85/P